A Nurse's Guide to

PCOS

DIET WITHOUT DEPRIVATION

Enjoy Your Favorite Foods

While Managing Symptoms, Boosting Fertility, and Embracing a Balanced Lifestyle

Giselle Wright, BSN RN

Giselle Wright, BSN RN
Binnovate Publishers

Table of Contents

Chapter 1

INTRODUCTION

Understanding PCOS

Polycystic Ovarian Syndrome (PCOS) is a common hormonal disorder that affects approximately 1 in 10 women of reproductive age. Characterized by a combination of symptoms, including irregular menstrual cycles, excess androgen levels, and polycystic ovaries, PCOS can lead to a range of health issues, including infertility, weight gain, and metabolic disorders.

The exact cause of PCOS is still not fully understood, but it is believed to be linked to insulin resistance, inflammation, and genetic factors. Women with PCOS often experience symptoms such as acne, excessive hair growth (hirsutism), and thinning hair, which can significantly impact their quality of life and emotional well-being.

The Importance of Nutrition

Nutrition plays a crucial role in managing PCOS symptoms and improving overall health. A well-balanced diet can help regulate insulin levels, support weight management, and promote hormonal balance. By focusing on nutrient-dense foods, women with PCOS can experience improvements in their symptoms and overall well-being.

Key nutritional strategies for managing PCOS include:

Emphasizing Whole Foods: Prioritizing whole, minimally processed foods such as fruits, vegetables, whole grains, lean proteins, and healthy fats can provide essential nutrients while helping to stabilize blood sugar levels.

Balancing Macronutrients: A balanced intake of carbohydrates, proteins, and fats is vital for managing insulin levels. Women with PCOS may benefit from a lower carbohydrate intake, focusing on complex carbohydrates that are high in fiber.

Incorporating Anti-Inflammatory Foods: Foods rich in antioxidants, omega-3 fatty acids, and anti-inflammatory compounds can help reduce inflammation and support hormonal balance. Examples include fatty fish, nuts, seeds, and colorful fruits and vegetables.

Staying Hydrated: Proper hydration is essential for overall health and can help manage cravings and support metabolic function.

The Philosophy of "Diet Without Deprivation"

The philosophy of "Diet Without Deprivation" emphasizes that managing PCOS does not mean giving up the foods you love or following a restrictive diet. Instead, it focuses on making mindful choices that allow for enjoyment and satisfaction while still promoting health and well-being.

Moderation Over Restriction: Rather than labeling foods as "good" or "bad," this approach encourages moderation. It's about finding a balance that allows you to enjoy your favorite foods while also making choices that support your health.

Smart Swaps: The concept of "Diet Without Deprivation" includes making smarter food swaps that can satisfy cravings without compromising health. For example, choosing whole grain options instead of refined grains, or using healthier fats in cooking.

Mindful Eating: Practicing mindful eating can help you develop a healthier relationship with food. This involves paying attention to hunger cues, savoring each bite, and enjoying the experience of eating without distractions.

Emotional Support: Managing PCOS can be challenging, and it's essential to address the emotional aspects of eating. This philosophy encourages self-compassion and understanding, reminding you that it's okay to indulge occasionally without guilt.

Chapter 2

My Personal Story (the Author)

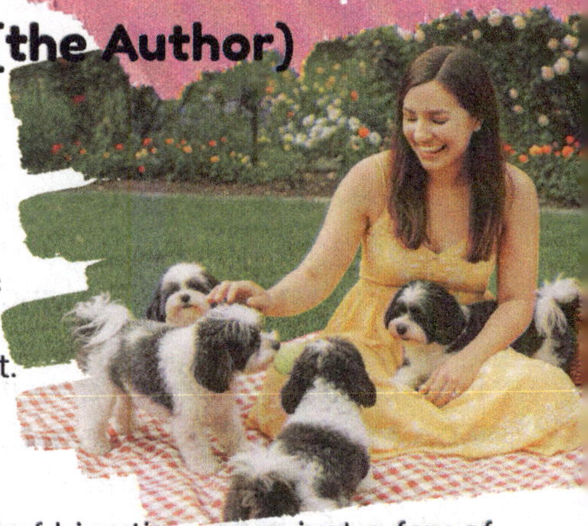

My Journey with PCOS

As a woman diagnosed with Polycystic Ovarian Syndrome (PCOS), my journey has been filled with challenges, learning experiences, and ultimately, empowerment. For five long years, I struggled with symptoms that left me feeling frustrated and confused. Irregular menstrual cycles, weight fluctuations, and the emotional toll of hirsutism were just a few of the hurdles I faced. I felt like I was on a rollercoaster, with no clear direction or understanding of what was happening to my body.

It wasn't until I began to take charge of my health that everything started to change. I immersed myself in research, seeking out information about PCOS and its management. I learned that nutrition plays a pivotal role in managing symptoms and improving overall health. This realization sparked a passion within me—a desire to not only heal myself but also to help other women facing similar struggles.

My Nursing Background

As a registered nurse, I have always been drawn to the field of healthcare. My nursing education provided me with a solid foundation in understanding the human body, disease processes, and the importance of holistic care. However, my personal experience with PCOS opened my eyes to the critical role that nutrition plays in health and wellness.

Through my nursing practice, I witnessed firsthand the impact of lifestyle choices on patients' health outcomes. I realized that many women, like myself, were not receiving the support they needed to manage their conditions effectively. This realization fueled my determination to bridge the gap between medical knowledge and practical nutrition advice.

My Passion for Nutrition

With my nursing background as a springboard, I pursued further education in nutrition, earning a certificate in Food and Nutrition Science from Stanford University. This journey deepened my understanding of how food affects our bodies, particularly in relation to hormonal balance and metabolic health.

I became passionate about creating a supportive environment for women with PCOS, where they could learn to embrace a balanced lifestyle without feeling deprived. I wanted to empower women to make informed choices about their nutrition, helping them to understand that they could enjoy their favorite foods while still managing their symptoms.

Embracing a Balanced Lifestyle

Through my research and personal experience, I developed the philosophy of "Diet Without Deprivation." I learned that it is possible to enjoy delicious meals while prioritizing health. This approach emphasizes moderation, smart swaps, and mindful eating, allowing women to cultivate a positive relationship with food.

As I continue my journey, I am committed to sharing my knowledge and experiences with others. I believe that by providing practical strategies, delicious recipes, and emotional support, we can create a community of women who are empowered to take charge of their health and fertility.

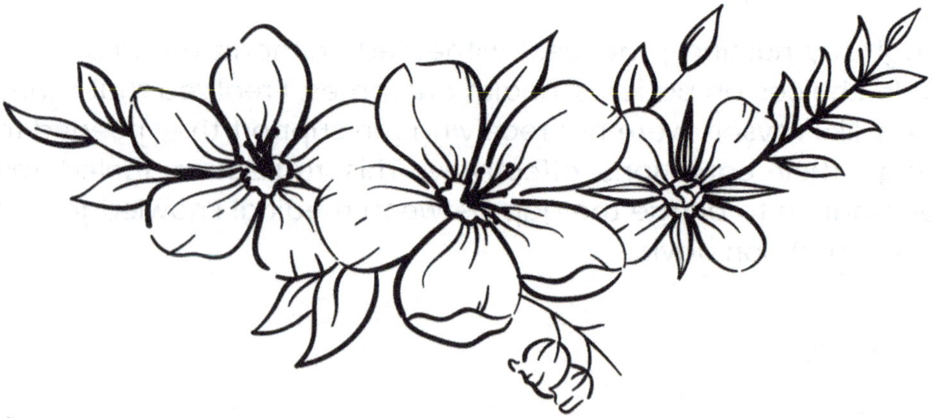

Chapter 3

The 80/20 Rule: Finding Balance

Understanding the 80/20 Rule

The 80/20 rule is a simple yet powerful concept that can transform the way you approach your diet and overall health. At its core, the 80/20 rule suggests that you should aim to consume healthy, nutrient-dense foods 80% of the time while allowing yourself the freedom to enjoy your favorite treats or less nutritious options 20% of the time. This approach promotes balance and sustainability, making it easier to maintain a healthy lifestyle without feeling deprived.

Why the 80/20 Rule Works

Flexibility: The 80/20 rule allows for flexibility in your eating habits. It acknowledges that life is about enjoyment, and food is a significant part of that experience. By allowing yourself to indulge occasionally, you can satisfy cravings without guilt, which can help prevent binge eating or feelings of deprivation.

Sustainability: Strict diets often lead to burnout and frustration. The 80/20 rule encourages a more sustainable approach to eating, making it easier to stick to healthy habits in the long run. It promotes a mindset of moderation rather than restriction.
Focus on Nutrient-Dense Foods: By prioritizing healthy foods 80% of the time, you ensure that your body receives the essential nutrients it needs to function optimally. This is especially important for women with PCOS, as proper nutrition can help manage symptoms and support hormonal balance.

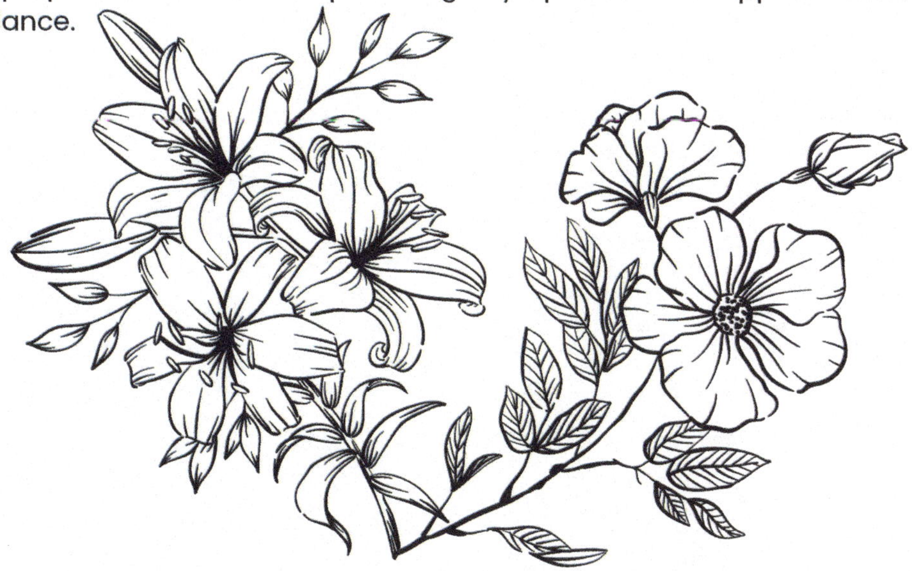

Applying the 80/20 Rule to Daily Eating Habits

Plan Your Meals: Start by planning your meals for the week. Aim to fill your plate with whole, nutrient-dense foods such as fruits, vegetables, lean proteins, whole grains, and healthy fats. This will make up the 80% of your diet.

Track Your Intake: Keep a food journal or use a tracking app to monitor your eating habits. This can help you identify areas where you may be leaning too heavily on less nutritious options and guide you toward a more balanced approach.

Mindful Indulgence: When it comes to the 20% of your diet, choose your indulgences wisely. Instead of mindlessly snacking on junk food, opt for treats that you genuinely enjoy. This could be a slice of cake at a celebration, a favorite dessert, or a savory dish you love. Savor each bite and enjoy the experience.

Be Flexible: Life is unpredictable, and there will be times when you may not stick to the 80/20 rule perfectly. That's okay! The key is to maintain a flexible mindset and return to your healthy habits when you can.
Celebrate Progress: Focus on the positive changes you're making rather than fixating on perfection. Celebrate your successes, whether it's trying a new healthy recipe or choosing a nutritious snack over a less healthy option.

Chapter 4

Smart Swaps for Everyday Foods

Making healthier choices doesn't have to mean sacrificing the foods you love. By incorporating smart swaps into your daily meals, you can enjoy your favorite dishes while still supporting your health and managing PCOS. This chapter will provide you with practical tips on how to replace common ingredients with healthier alternatives, helping you to create balanced meals that nourish your body and satisfy your cravings.

White Rice → Cauliflower Rice

Why: Cauliflower rice is low in carbohydrates and calories while being high in fiber and nutrients. It can help regulate blood sugar levels and is a great alternative for those managing PCOS.

How to Use: Simply pulse cauliflower florets in a food processor until they resemble rice, then sauté or steam until tender.

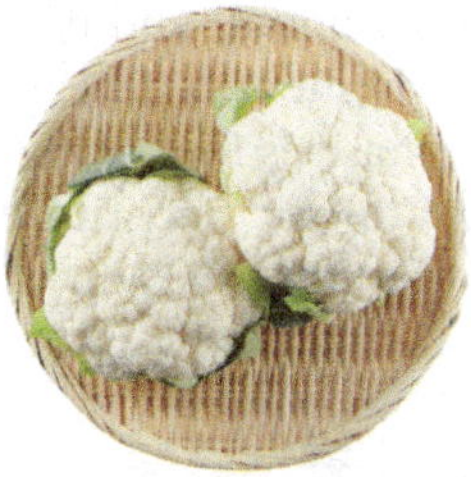

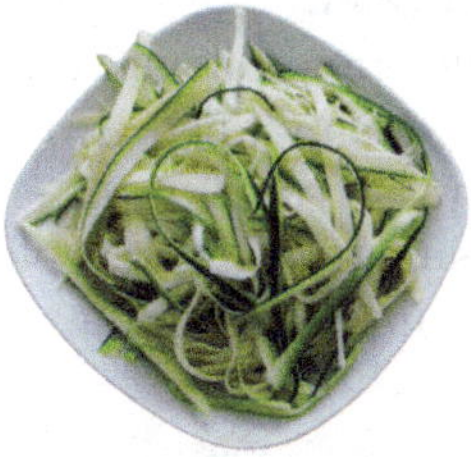

Regular Pasta → Zucchini Noodles or Whole Grain Pasta

Why: Zucchini noodles (zoodles) are low in carbs and calories, while whole grain pasta offers more fiber and nutrients than traditional pasta.

How to Use: Spiralize zucchini into noodles and sauté briefly, or choose whole grain pasta for a more filling option.

Sugar → Natural Sweeteners (like Stevia or Monk Fruit)

Why: Natural sweeteners have little to no calories and do not spike blood sugar levels, making them a better choice for women with PCOS.

How to Use: Use in baking, beverages, or as a sweetener for yogurt and oatmeal.

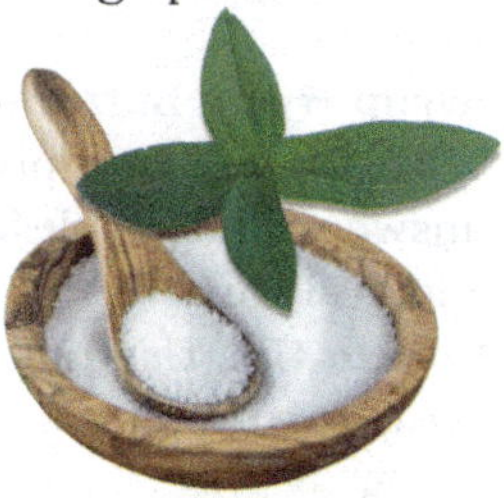

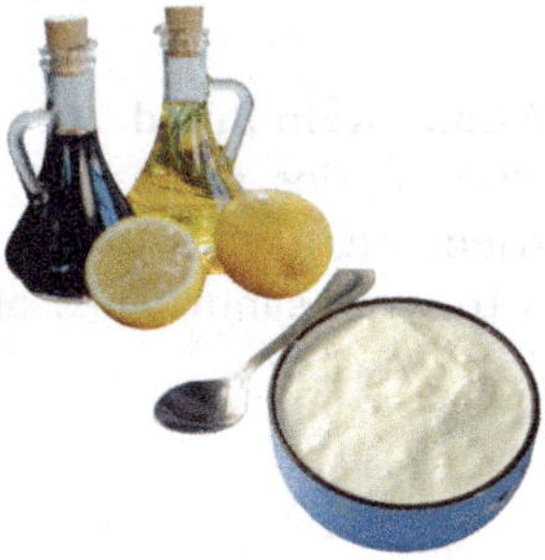

Creamy Dressings → Olive Oil and Vinegar or Greek Yogurt Dressing

Why: Creamy dressings can be high in unhealthy fats and calories. Olive oil and vinegar provide healthy fats and flavor without the extra calories.

How to Use: Mix olive oil with balsamic vinegar, lemon juice, or herbs for a light dressing, or use Greek yogurt as a base for a creamy dressing.

Potato Chips → Air-Popped Popcorn or Veggie Chips

Why: Air-popped popcorn is a whole grain, low-calorie snack that can satisfy crunch cravings without the unhealthy fats found in potato chips.

How to Use: Season air-popped popcorn with your favorite spices or opt for baked veggie chips for a healthier crunch.

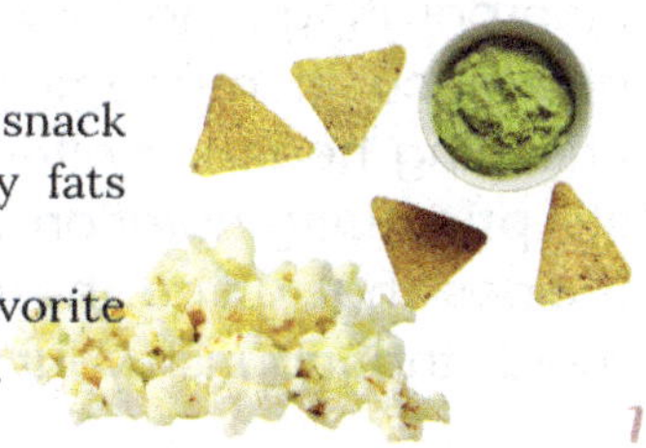

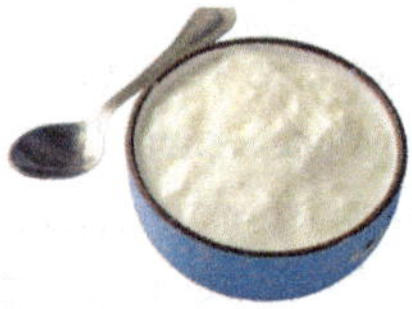

Regular Yogurt ➜ Greek Yogurt or Coconut Yogurt
Why: Greek yogurt is higher in protein and lower in sugar than regular yogurt, making it a better choice for managing cravings and promoting satiety.
How to Use: Use Greek yogurt in smoothies, parfaits, or as a base for dressings and dips.

Regular Flour ➜ Almond Flour or Coconut Flour
Why: Almond and coconut flours are lower in carbohydrates and higher in fiber and healthy fats, making them great alternatives for baking.
How to Use: Substitute regular flour with almond or coconut flour in recipes, adjusting liquid ingredients as needed.

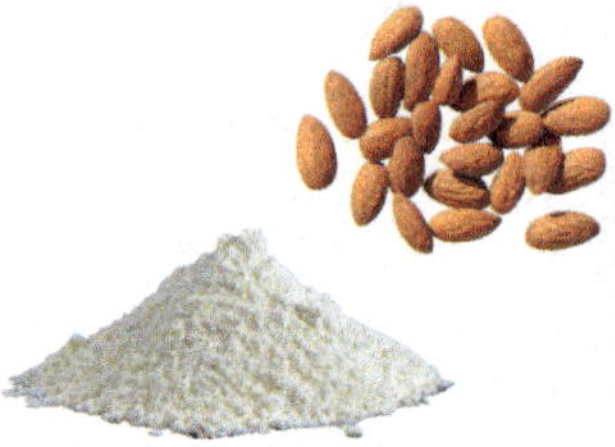

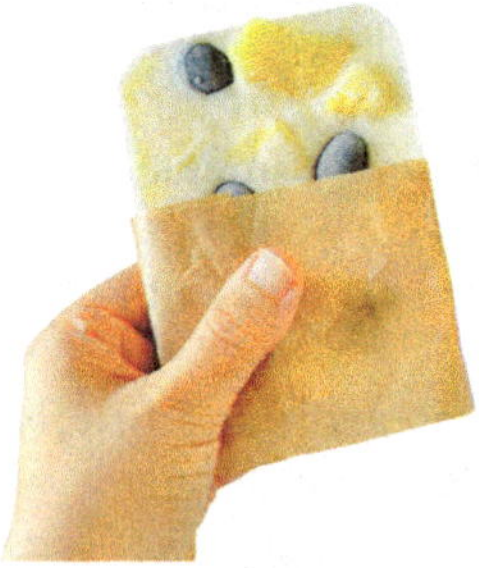

Ice Cream ➜ Frozen Yogurt or Banana Ice Cream
Why: Frozen yogurt is lower in calories and sugar than traditional ice cream, while banana ice cream (made from blended frozen bananas) is a healthy, creamy alternative.
How to Use: Blend frozen bananas until smooth for a simple, healthy dessert, or choose a low-sugar frozen yogurt option.

Syrup ➜ Nut Butter or Unsweetened Applesauce
Why: Nut butter provides healthy fats and protein, while unsweetened applesauce adds natural sweetness without added sugars.
How to Use: Use nut butter on pancakes or toast, or replace syrup with applesauce in baking.

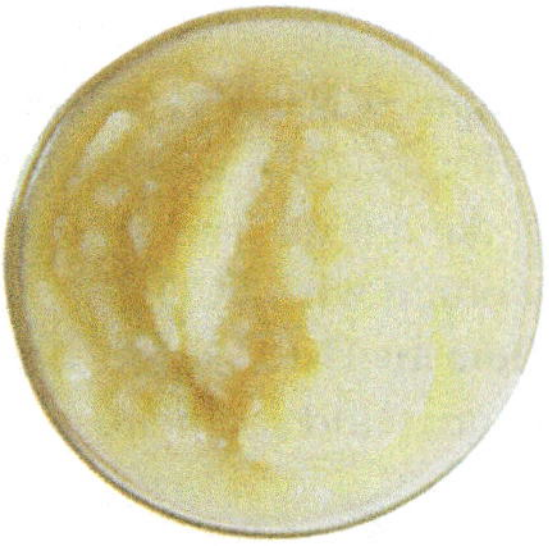

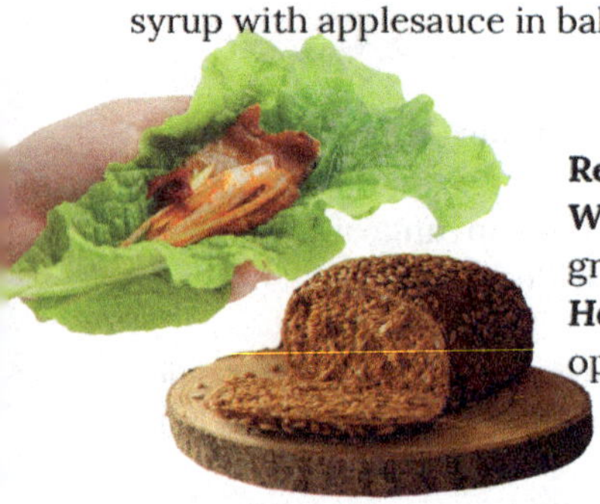

Regular Bread ➜ Lettuce Wraps or Whole Grain Bread
Why: Lettuce wraps are low in carbs and calories, while whole grain bread offers more fiber and nutrients than white bread.
How to Use: Use large lettuce leaves to wrap sandwiches or opt for whole grain bread for toast and sandwiches.

Incorporating smart swaps into your daily meals can make a significant difference in managing PCOS and supporting your overall health. By choosing healthier alternatives, you can enjoy your favorite foods while still prioritizing nutrition. In the following chapters, we will explore delicious recipes that utilize these smart swaps, helping you to create satisfying meals that nourish your body and support your journey.

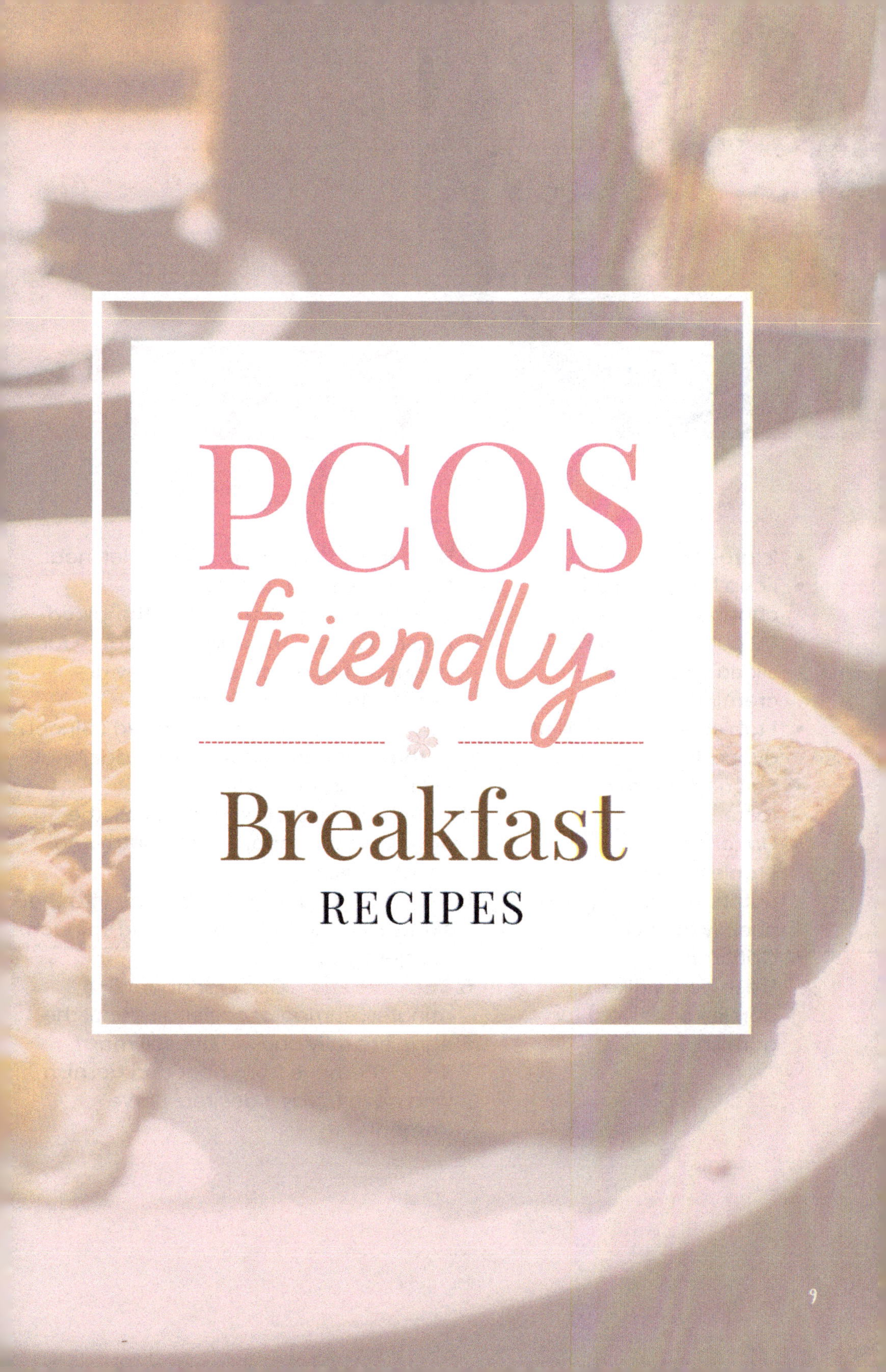

PCOS *friendly*

Breakfast RECIPES

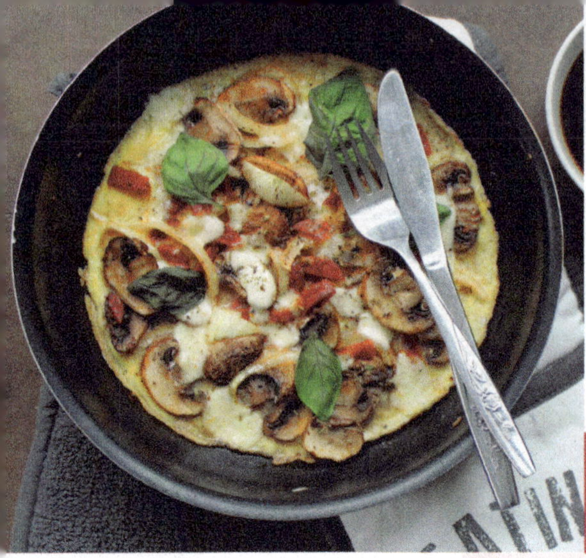

Savory Spinach and Mushroom Egg Scramble

SERVING SIZE
Serves 1

INGREDIENTS

- 2 large eggs
- 1 cup fresh spinach, chopped
- 1/2 cup mushrooms, sliced (button or cremini)
- 1 tablespoon olive oil or avocado oil
- Salt and pepper to taste
- *Optional* 1 tablespoon nutritional yeast (for a cheesy flavor)
- *Optional* Fresh herbs (like parsley or chives) for garnish

DIRECTIONS

1. **Heat the Oil:** In a non-stick skillet, heat the olive oil over medium heat.
2. **Sauté the Mushrooms:** Add the sliced mushrooms to the skillet and sauté for about 3-4 minutes, or until they are tender and lightly browned.
3. **Add Spinach:** Add the chopped spinach to the skillet and cook for an additional 1-2 minutes, until wilted.
4. **Whisk the Eggs:** In a bowl, whisk the eggs with salt, pepper, and nutritional yeast (if using).
5. **Combine:** Pour the egg mixture into the skillet with the mushrooms and spinach. Stir gently to combine.
6. **Cook the Eggs:** Cook for about 3-4 minutes, stirring occasionally, until the eggs are fully cooked but still moist.
7. **Serve:** Remove from heat and garnish with fresh herbs if desired. Serve immediately

Nutrition Information (Per Serving)

Calories	250
Protein	18g
Carbohydrates	6g
Dietary Fiber	2g
Sugars	1g
Fat	18g
Saturated Fat	3g

"You are enough."

QUICK NOTES

TIPS FOR CUSTOMIZATION

- **Add Protein:** For extra protein, consider adding cooked chicken, turkey bacon, or tofu.
- **Spice it Up:** Add a pinch of red pepper flakes or hot sauce for a kick.
- **Vegetable Variations:** Feel free to include other vegetables like bell peppers, onions, or zucchini.

Why is this recipe good for PCOS?

This Savory Spinach and Mushroom Egg Scramble is rich in protein and healthy fats, which help regulate blood sugar levels and promote satiety. The combination of spinach and mushrooms provides essential vitamins and minerals while being low in carbohydrates, making it an excellent choice for managing PCOS symptoms. Additionally, the healthy fats from olive oil support hormone balance, which is crucial for women with PCOS.

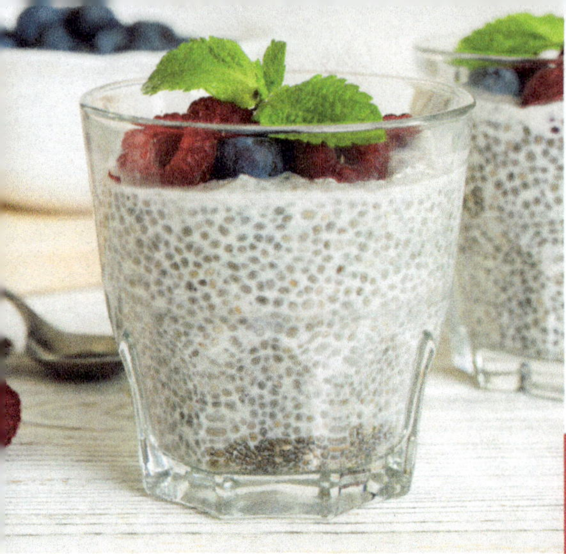

Chia Seed Pudding with Almond Milk and Berries

SERVING SIZE
Serves 1

INGREDIENTS

- 1/4 cup chia seeds
- 1 cup unsweetened almond milk
- 1 tablespoon maple syrup or a low-carb sweetener (like stevia or monk fruit) to taste
- 1/2 teaspoon vanilla extract
- 1/2 cup mixed berries (strawberries, blueberries, raspberries)
- *Optional* 1 tablespoon almond butter or coconut flakes for topping

DIRECTIONS

1. **Mix Ingredients:** In a bowl or jar, combine chia seeds, almond milk, maple syrup (or sweetener), and vanilla extract. Stir well to ensure the chia seeds are evenly distributed.
2. **Refrigerate:** Cover the bowl or jar and refrigerate for at least 4 hours or overnight. The chia seeds will absorb the liquid and thicken to a pudding-like consistency.
3. **Stir and Serve:** After chilling, stir the pudding to break up any clumps. Top with mixed berries and optional almond butter or coconut flakes before serving.

Nutrition Information (Per Serving)

Calories	250
Protein	6g
Carbohydrates	20g
Dietary Fiber	15g
Sugars	5g
Fat	16g
Saturated Fat	1g

"Believe in your strength."

QUICK NOTES

TIPS FOR CUSTOMIZATION

- **Flavor Variations:** Add a pinch of cinnamon or cocoa powder for different flavor profiles.
- **Fruit Options:** Use any seasonal fruits or your favorite berries for topping.
- **Nut Milk Alternatives:** Substitute almond milk with coconut milk or any other dairy-free milk of your choice.

Why is this recipe good for PCOS?

Chia seeds are an excellent source of omega-3 fatty acids, fiber, and protein, which help regulate blood sugar levels and promote satiety. The high fiber content aids in digestion and can help manage weight, which is beneficial for women with PCOS. Almond milk is low in carbohydrates and calories, making this pudding a nutritious and satisfying breakfast or snack option that supports overall hormonal balance.

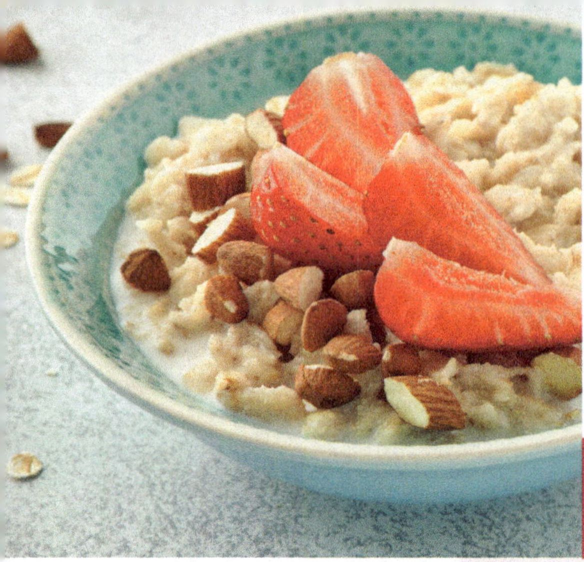

Quinoa Breakfast Bowl with Almonds and Sliced Strawberries

SERVING SIZE
Serves 1

INGREDIENTS

- 1/2 cup cooked quinoa (preferably chilled)
- 1/2 cup unsweetened almond milk
- 1 tablespoon almond butter or chopped almonds
- 1/2 teaspoon cinnamon
- 1 tablespoon maple syrup or a low-carb sweetener (like stevia or monkfruit) to taste
- 1/2 cup fresh strawberries, sliced
- *Optional*
  1 tablespoon chia seeds or hemp seeds for added nutrition

DIRECTIONS

1. **Prepare Quinoa:** If you haven't already, cook quinoa according to package instructions. Allow it to cool or use chilled quinoa for a refreshing breakfast.
2. **Mix Ingredients:** In a bowl, combine the cooked quinoa, almond milk, almond butter (or chopped almonds), cinnamon, and maple syrup (or sweetener). Stir until well combined.
3. **Top with Strawberries:** Add the sliced strawberries on top of the quinoa mixture. If desired, sprinkle with chia seeds or hemp seeds for extra nutrition.
4. **Serve:** Enjoy immediately as a nutritious breakfast or snack.

Nutrition Information (Per Serving)

Calories	350
Protein	10g
Carbohydrates	40g
Dietary Fiber	8g
Sugars	8g
Fat	16g
Saturated Fat	1g

"Embrace your journey."

QUICK NOTES

TIPS FOR CUSTOMIZATION

- **Nut Variations:** Substitute almonds with walnuts, pecans, or any nut of your choice.
- **Fruit Options:** Use other berries or fruits like blueberries, raspberries, or banana slices.
- **Add Protein:** Mix in a scoop of protein powder for an extra protein boost.

Why is this recipe good for PCOS?

Quinoa is a complete protein and a great source of fiber, which helps regulate blood sugar levels and promotes satiety. The healthy fats from almond butter and almonds support hormone balance, while the strawberries provide antioxidants and vitamins. This breakfast bowl is low in refined sugars and high in nutrients, making it an excellent choice for women managing PCOS.

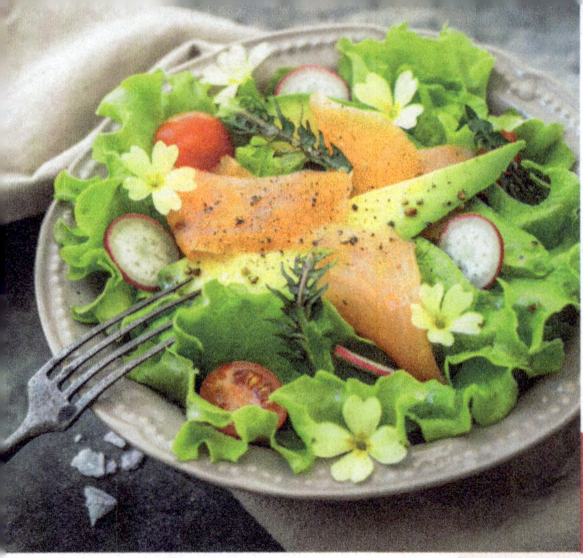

Avocado and Smoked Salmon Lettuce Wraps

SERVING SIZE
Serves 1

INGREDIENTS

- 4 large lettuce leaves (such as romaine or butter lettuce)
- 1 ripe avocado, sliced
- 4 ounces smoked salmon
- 1/4 small red onion, thinly sliced
  1 tablespoon capers (optional)
- Juice of 1/2 lemon
- Salt and pepper to taste
- *Optional*
  Fresh dill or chives for garnish

DIRECTIONS

1. **Prepare Lettuce Leaves:** Carefully wash and dry the lettuce leaves. Set aside.
2. **Assemble Wraps:** On each lettuce leaf, layer slices of avocado and smoked salmon.
3. **Add Toppings:** Top with thinly sliced red onion and capers (if using). Squeeze fresh lemon juice over the top and season with salt and pepper to taste.
4. **Garnish:** If desired, sprinkle with fresh dill or chives for added flavor.
5. **Serve:** Enjoy immediately as a light and nutritious breakfast or snack.

Nutrition Information (Per Serving)

Calories	300
Protein	20g
Carbohydrates	10g
Dietary Fiber	7g
Sugars	1g
Fat	22g
Saturated Fat	3g

"You are powerful beyond measure."

QUICK NOTES

TIPS FOR CUSTOMIZATION

- **Add Veggies:** Include additional toppings like cucumber slices, radishes, or bell peppers for extra crunch and nutrients.
- **Spice it Up:** Add a dash of hot sauce or red pepper flakes for a spicy kick.
- **Swap Proteins:** Substitute smoked salmon with canned tuna or grilled chicken for variety.

Why is this recipe good for PCOS?

Avocado is rich in healthy fats and fiber, which help regulate blood sugar levels and promote satiety. Smoked salmon provides high-quality protein and omega-3 fatty acids, which are beneficial for hormone balance. This recipe is low in carbohydrates and packed with nutrients, making it an excellent choice for women managing PCOS while enjoying a delicious and satisfying meal.

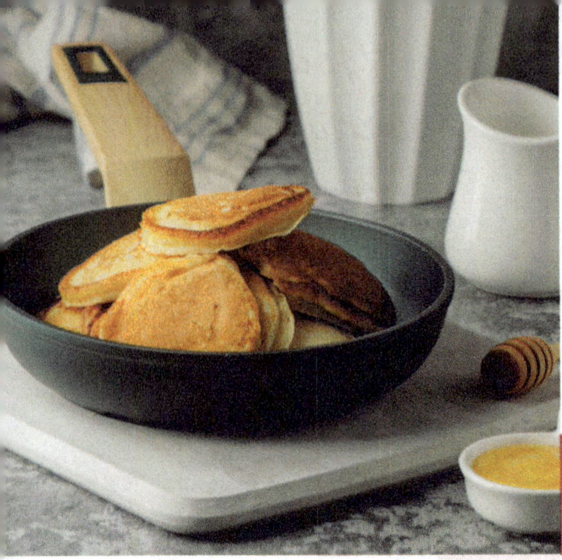

Coconut Flour Pancakes with Sugar-Free Maple Syrup

SERVING SIZE
Serves 1 (makes about 2-3 pancakes)

INGREDIENTS

- 1/4 cup coconut flour
- 1/4 teaspoon baking powder
- 1/4 teaspoon salt
- 3 large eggs
- 1/4 cup unsweetened almond milk (or any dairy-free milk)
- 1 tablespoon coconut oil, melted (plus extra for cooking)
- 1 teaspoon vanilla extract
- *Optional* Sugar-free maple syrup for serving

DIRECTIONS

1. **Mix Dry Ingredients:** In a bowl, combine coconut flour, baking powder, and salt. Mix well to ensure there are no lumps.
2. **Combine Wet Ingredients:** In a separate bowl, whisk together the eggs, almond milk, melted coconut oil, and vanilla extract until smooth.
3. **Combine Mixtures:** Gradually add the wet ingredients to the dry ingredients, stirring until well combined. Let the batter sit for about 5 minutes to thicken.
4. **Cook Pancakes:** Heat a non-stick skillet over medium heat and add a small amount of coconut oil. Pour about 1/4 cup of batter onto the skillet for each pancake. Cook for 2-3 minutes, or until bubbles form on the surface, then flip and cook for an additional 1-2 minutes until golden brown.
5. **Serve:** Stack the pancakes on a plate and serve warm with sugar-free maple syrup, if desired.

Nutrition Information (Per Serving)

Calories	300
Protein	12g
Carbohydrates	20g
Dietary Fiber	10g
Sugars	2g
Fat	20g
Saturated Fat	10g

"Your voice matters."

QUICK NOTES

TIPS FOR CUSTOMIZATION

- **Add Flavor:** Mix in cinnamon or nutmeg for added flavor.
- **Fruit Toppings:** Top with fresh berries or sliced bananas for natural sweetness.
- **Nut Variations:** Add chopped nuts or seeds to the batter for extra crunch.

Why is this recipe good for PCOS?

Coconut flour is high in fiber and low in carbohydrates, making it a great option for managing blood sugar levels. The healthy fats from coconut oil and the protein from eggs help promote satiety and hormone balance. This pancake recipe is a delicious, low-carb alternative to traditional pancakes, allowing women with PCOS to enjoy a satisfying breakfast without the guilt.

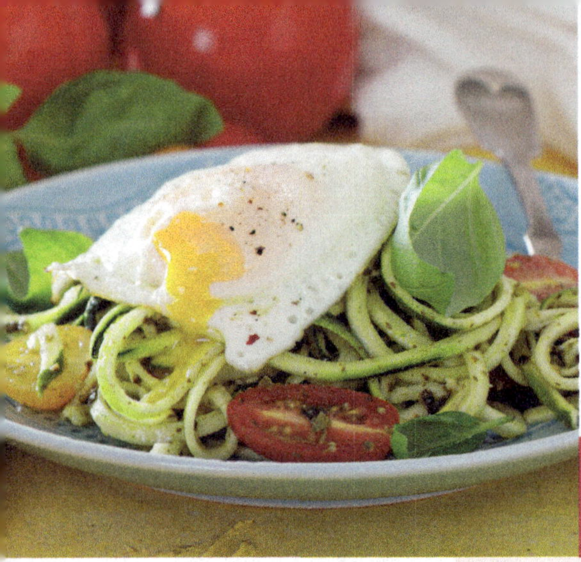

Zucchini Noodles with Scrambled Eggs and Cherry Tomatoes

SERVING SIZE
Serves 1

INGREDIENTS

- 2 medium zucchinis, spiralized into noodles
- 2 large eggs
- 1 cup cherry tomatoes, halved
- 1 tablespoon olive oil
- 1 clove garlic, minced
- Salt and pepper to taste
- *Optional* Fresh basil or parsley for garnish
- *Optional* Nutritional yeast for a cheesy flavor

DIRECTIONS

1. **Prepare Zucchini Noodles:** Spiralize the zucchinis into noodles and set aside.
2. **Sauté Garlic and Tomatoes:** In a large skillet, heat olive oil over medium heat. Add minced garlic and sauté for about 30 seconds until fragrant. Add the halved cherry tomatoes and cook for 2-3 minutes until they start to soften.
3. **Add Zucchini Noodles:** Add the spiralized zucchini noodles to the skillet and cook for an additional 2-3 minutes, stirring gently until the noodles are tender but still slightly crisp.
4. **Scramble the Eggs:** In a bowl, whisk the eggs with salt and pepper. Push the zucchini noodles and tomatoes to one side of the skillet and pour the eggs into the other side. Scramble the eggs until fully cooked, then mix them with the zucchini noodles and tomatoes.
5. **Serve:** Remove from heat and garnish with fresh herbs and nutritional yeast if desired. Serve immediately.

Nutrition Information (Per Serving)

Calories	250
Protein	12g
Carbohydrates	10g
Dietary Fiber	4g
Sugars	4g
Fat	20g
Saturated Fat	3g

"Shine your light."

QUICK NOTES

TIPS FOR CUSTOMIZATION

- **Add Protein:** Include cooked chicken, turkey, or tofu for extra protein.
- **Spice it Up:** Add red pepper flakes or hot sauce for a spicy kick.
- **Vegetable Variations:** Incorporate other vegetables like bell peppers, spinach, or onions for added nutrition.

Why is this recipe good for PCOS?

Zucchini noodles are low in carbohydrates and high in fiber, making them an excellent choice for managing blood sugar levels. The combination of eggs provides high-quality protein and healthy fats, which are essential for hormone balance. This dish is nutrient-dense and satisfying, making it a great option for women with PCOS looking for a healthy and delicious meal.

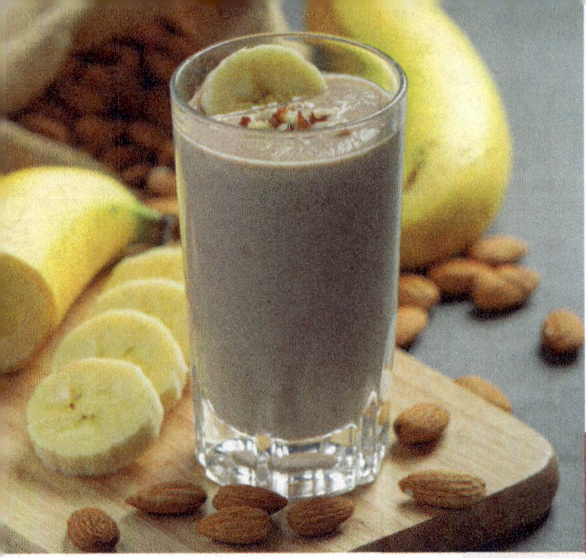

Almond Butter and Banana Smoothie

SERVING SIZE
Serves 1

INGREDIENTS

- 1 medium ripe banana
- 2 tablespoons almond butter
- 1 cup unsweetened almond milk
- 1 tablespoon chia seeds (optional)
- 1/2 teaspoon cinnamon (optional)
- Ice cubes (optional, for a chilled smoothie)

DIRECTIONS

1. **Combine Ingredients:** In a blender, add the banana, almond butter, unsweetened almond milk, chia seeds (if using), and cinnamon (if using).
2. **Blend:** Blend on high speed until smooth and creamy. If you prefer a thicker smoothie, add a few ice cubes and blend again until desired consistency is reached.
3. **Serve:** Pour the smoothie into a glass and enjoy immediately.

Nutrition Information (Per Serving)

Calories	350
Protein	10g
Carbohydrates	30g
Dietary Fiber	8g
Sugars	12g
Fat	22g
Saturated Fat	2g

"Dream big, act bold."

QUICK NOTES

TIPS FOR CUSTOMIZATION

- **Add Greens:** Toss in a handful of spinach or kale for added nutrients without altering the flavor significantly.
- **Protein Boost:** Add a scoop of protein powder for an extra protein boost.
- **Flavor Variations:** Experiment with different nut butters, such as cashew or peanut butter, for variety.

Why is this recipe good for PCOS?

This smoothie is rich in healthy fats from almond butter, which helps regulate blood sugar levels and promotes satiety. The banana provides natural sweetness and potassium, while chia seeds add fiber and omega-3 fatty acids, which are beneficial for hormone balance. This nutrient-dense smoothie is a quick and easy breakfast option for women managing PCOS, providing sustained energy throughout the morning.

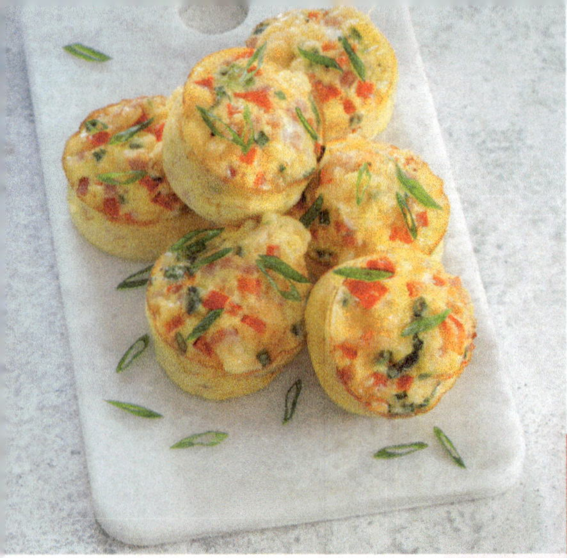

Egg Muffins with Spinach, Bell Peppers, and Turkey Bacon

SERVING SIZE
Serves 3 (2 muffins per serving)

INGREDIENTS

- 6 large eggs
- 1/2 cup unsweetened almond milk
- 1 cup fresh spinach, chopped
- 1/2 cup bell peppers, diced (any color)
- 4 slices turkey bacon, cooked and crumbled
- Salt and pepper to taste
- *Optional*
  1/4 teaspoon garlic powder or onion powder for added flavor

DIRECTIONS

1. **Preheat Oven:** Preheat your oven to 350°F (175°C). Grease a muffin tin with cooking spray or line with silicone muffin cups.
2. **Prepare Egg Mixture:** In a large bowl, whisk together the eggs and almond milk. Season with salt, pepper, and optional garlic or onion powder.
3. **Add Vegetables and Bacon:** Stir in the chopped spinach, diced bell peppers, and crumbled turkey bacon until evenly distributed.
4. **Fill Muffin Tin:** Pour the egg mixture evenly into the prepared muffin tin, filling each cup about 3/4 full.
5. **Bake:** Bake in the preheated oven for 18-20 minutes, or until the egg muffins are set and lightly golden on top.
6. **Cool and Serve:** Allow the muffins to cool for a few minutes before removing them from the tin. Serve warm or store in the refrigerator for later.

Nutrition Information (Per Serving)

Calories	200
Protein	18g
Carbohydrates	6g
Dietary Fiber	2g
Sugars	2g
Fat	12g
Saturated Fat	3g

"You are unstoppable."

QUICK NOTES

TIPS FOR CUSTOMIZATION

- **Add Cheese:** For a dairy-free option, use nutritional yeast for a cheesy flavor without the dairy.
- **Vegetable Variations:** Substitute or add other vegetables like zucchini, mushrooms, or onions for variety.
- **Herbs and Spices:** Experiment with fresh herbs like basil or cilantro for added flavor.

Why is this recipe good for PCOS?

These egg muffins are high in protein and healthy fats, which help regulate blood sugar levels and promote satiety. The combination of spinach and bell peppers provides essential vitamins and minerals, while turkey bacon adds lean protein without excess fat. This recipe is low in carbohydrates and can be made in advance, making it a convenient and nutritious option for women managing PCOS.

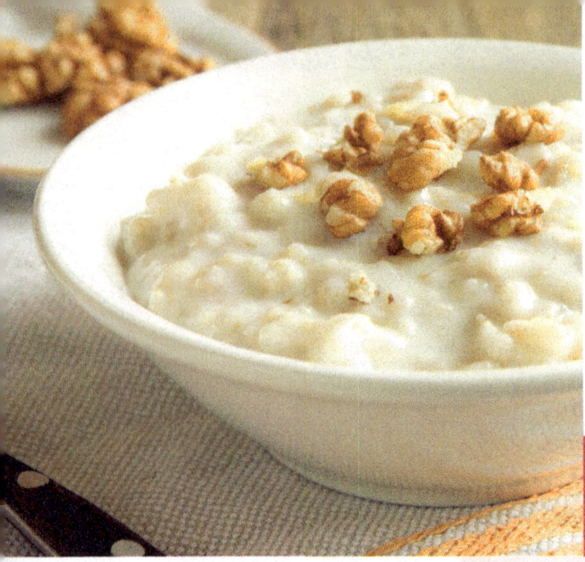

Flaxseed Meal Porridge with Cinnamon and Walnuts

SERVING SIZE
Serves 1

INGREDIENTS

- 1/4 cup ground flaxseed meal
- 1 cup unsweetened almond milk (or any dairy-free milk)
- 1/2 teaspoon cinnamon
- 1 tablespoon walnuts, chopped
- 1 tablespoon chia seeds (optional)
- 1 tablespoon maple syrup or a low-carb sweetener (like stevia or monk fruit) to taste
- *Optional*
  Fresh berries or sliced banana for topping

DIRECTIONS

1. **Combine Ingredients:** In a small saucepan, combine the ground flaxseed meal, almond milk, cinnamon, and chia seeds (if using). Stir well to combine.
2. **Cook the Porridge:** Heat the mixture over medium heat, stirring frequently, until it begins to thicken and bubble, about 3-5 minutes.
3. **Sweeten:** Once thickened, remove from heat and stir in the maple syrup or sweetener to taste.
4. **Serve:** Pour the porridge into a bowl and top with chopped walnuts and optional fresh berries or banana slices.

Nutrition Information (Per Serving)

Calories	300
Protein	10g
Carbohydrates	20g
Dietary Fiber	15g
Sugars	2g
Fat	22g
Saturated Fat	2g

"Strength comes from within."

QUICK NOTES

TIPS FOR CUSTOMIZATION

- **Nut Variations:** Substitute walnuts with pecans, almonds, or any nut of your choice.
- **Flavor Additions:** Add a splash of vanilla extract or a pinch of nutmeg for extra flavor.
- **Fruit Options:** Top with your favorite fruits, such as apples, pears, or berries, for added sweetness and nutrients.

Why is this recipe good for PCOS?

Flaxseed meal is rich in omega-3 fatty acids, fiber, and lignans, which can help regulate hormones and improve insulin sensitivity. The high fiber content aids in digestion and promotes satiety, making it beneficial for weight management. This porridge is low in carbohydrates and packed with nutrients, making it an excellent choice for women managing PCOS while enjoying a warm and comforting breakfast.

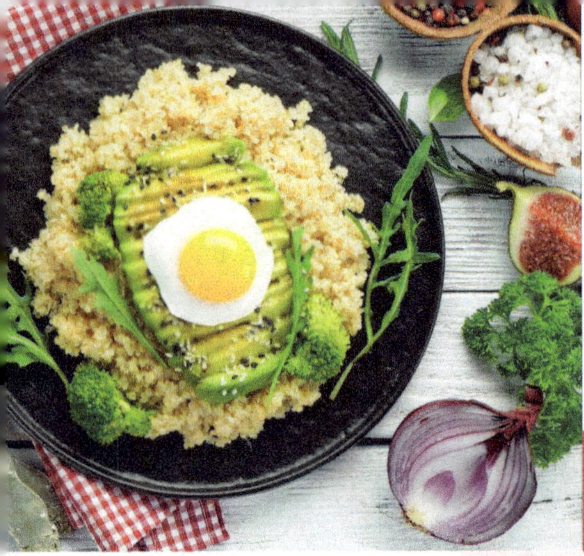

Cauliflower Rice Breakfast Bowl with Avocado and Poached Egg

SERVING SIZE
Serves 1

INGREDIENTS

- 1 cup cauliflower rice (fresh or frozen)
- 1 tablespoon olive oil
- 1/2 avocado, sliced
- 1 large egg
- Salt and pepper to taste
- *Optional*
  Fresh herbs (like cilantro or parsley) for garnish
- *Optional*
  Red pepper flakes for added spice

DIRECTIONS

1. **Cook Cauliflower Rice:** In a skillet, heat olive oil over medium heat. Add the cauliflower rice and sauté for about 5-7 minutes, stirring occasionally, until tender. Season with salt and pepper to taste.
2. **Poach the Egg:** While the cauliflower rice is cooking, bring a small pot of water to a gentle simmer. Crack the egg into a small bowl, then gently slide it into the simmering water. Poach for about 3-4 minutes, or until the white is set but the yolk is still runny. Remove with a slotted spoon and drain on a paper towel.
3. **Assemble the Bowl:** In a serving bowl, layer the cooked cauliflower rice, sliced avocado, and the poached egg on top.
4. **Garnish and Serve:** Sprinkle with fresh herbs and red pepper flakes if desired. Serve immediately.

Nutrition Information (Per Serving)

Calories	350
Protein	12g
Carbohydrates	15g
Dietary Fiber	8g
Sugars	2g
Fat	28g
Saturated Fat	4g

"Own your story."

QUICK NOTES

TIPS FOR CUSTOMIZATION

- **Add Veggies:** Incorporate other vegetables like spinach, bell peppers, or tomatoes for added nutrition.
- **Flavor Boost:** Drizzle with hot sauce or a squeeze of lemon juice for extra flavor.
- **Protein Variations:** Substitute the poached egg with scrambled eggs or a fried egg if preferred.

Why is this recipe good for PCOS?

This breakfast bowl is low in carbohydrates and high in healthy fats from avocado, which helps regulate blood sugar levels and promotes satiety. Cauliflower rice is a low-calorie, nutrient-dense alternative to traditional grains, providing fiber and vitamins. The poached egg adds high-quality protein, which is essential for hormone balance. This dish is a delicious and satisfying way to start the day while managing PCOS.

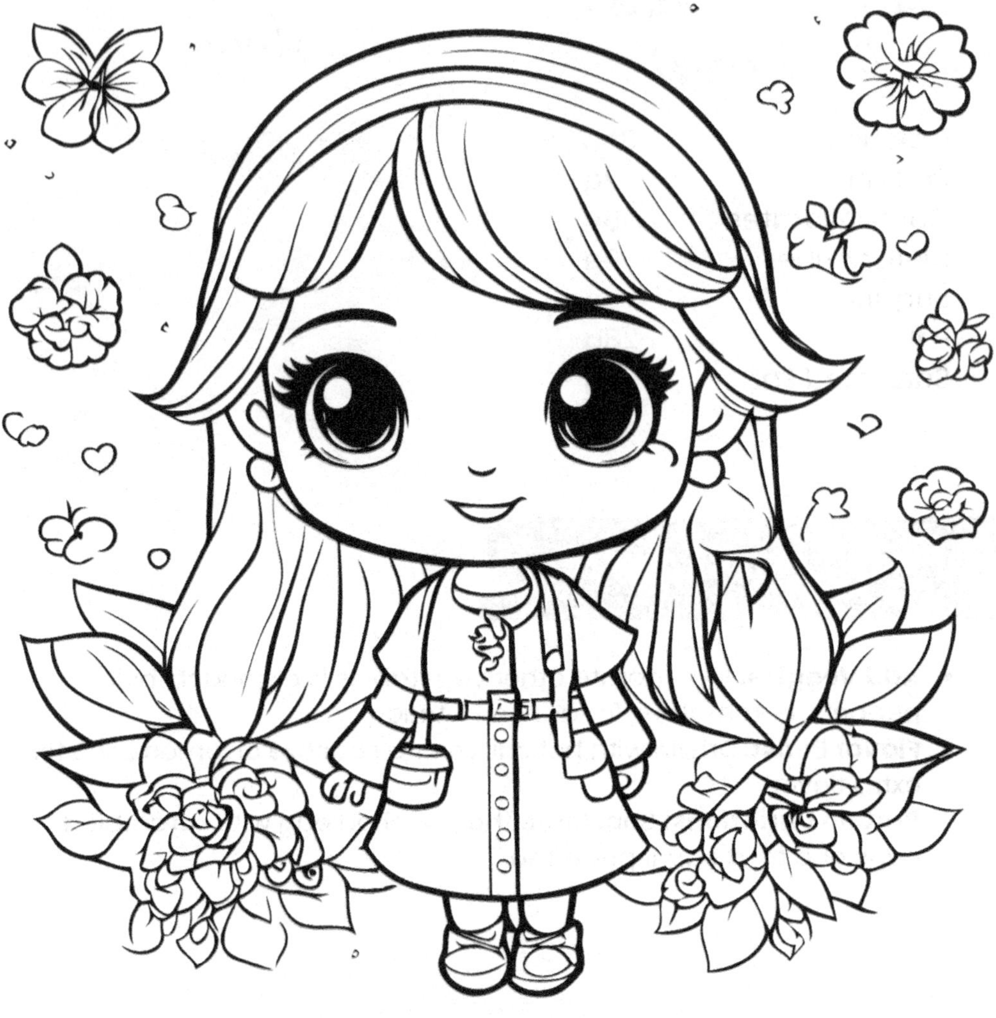

Hello, there! I hope you find these coloring pages fun. I deliberately included these here. I don't draw well, but I find comfort and a sense of relaxation when coloring easy drawings like this one. Allow me also to share a little bit about myself in these few coloring pages that I've added to this book. - G.

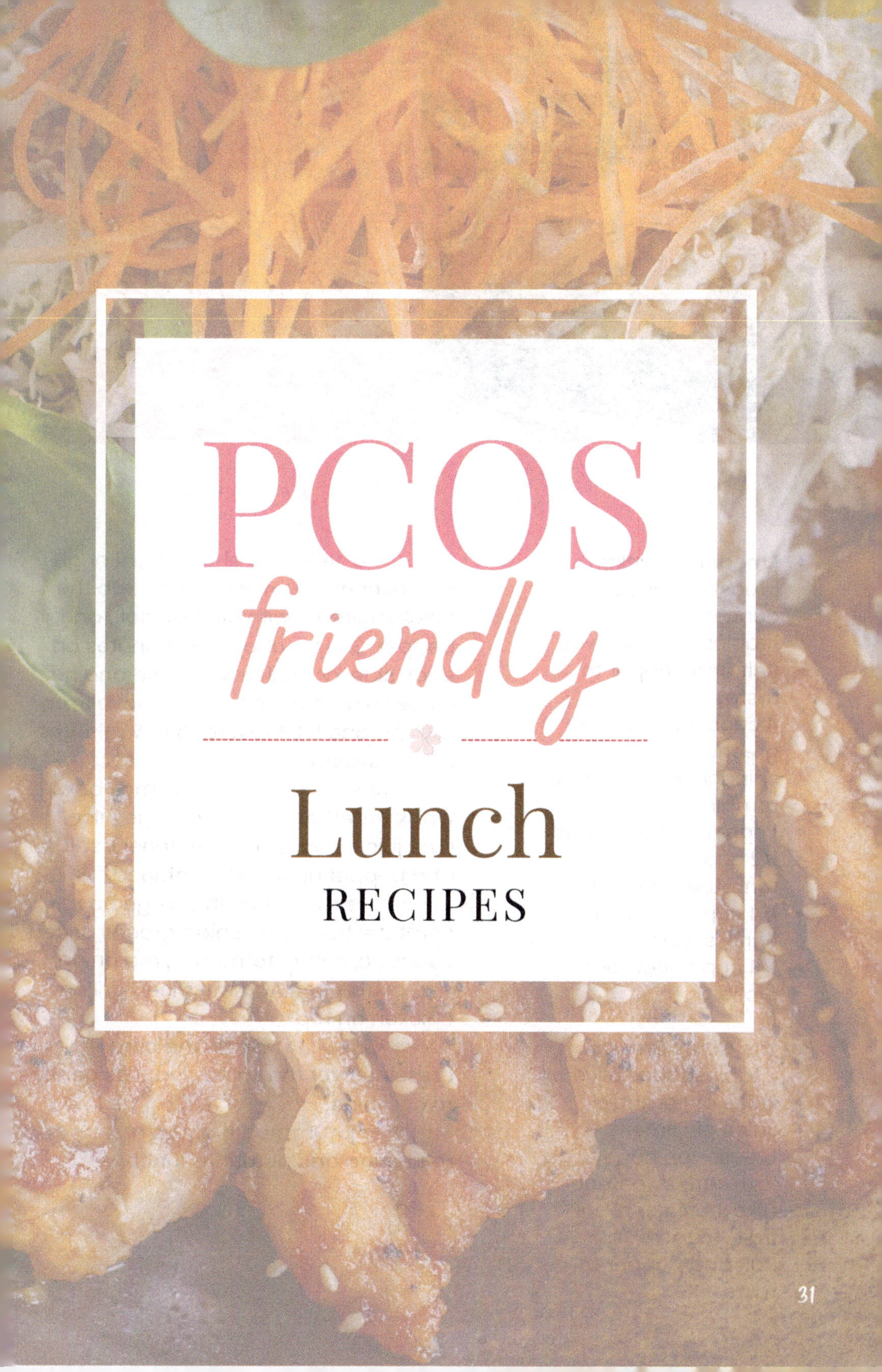

PCOS *friendly*

Lunch
RECIPES

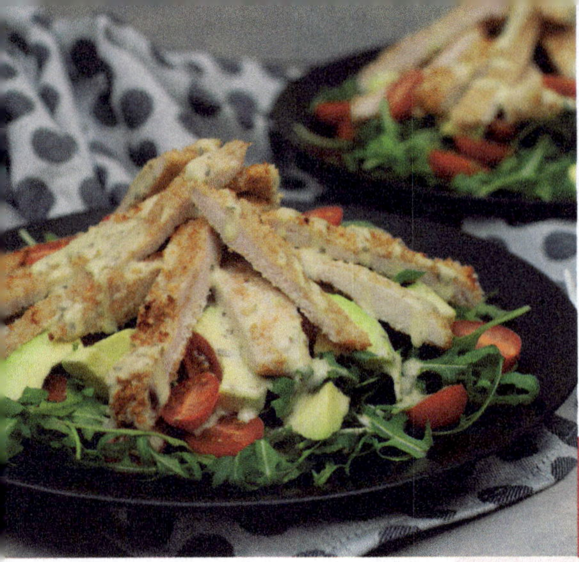

Grilled Chicken Salad with Avocado and Citrus Dressing

SERVING SIZE
Serves 1

INGREDIENTS

- 1 medium chicken breast (about 6 ounces)
- 1 tablespoon olive oil
- Salt and pepper to taste
- 4 cups mixed salad greens (such as spinach, arugula, and romaine)
- 1 ripe avocado, sliced
- 1/2 cup cherry tomatoes, halved
- 1/4 cup red onion, thinly sliced
- 1/4 cup cucumber, diced

For the Citrus Dressing

- 2 tablespoons olive oil
- Juice of 1 orange
- Juice of 1 lime
  1 teaspoon honey or a low-carb sweetener (like stevia or monk fruit) to taste
- Salt and pepper to taste

DIRECTIONS

1. **Grill the Chicken:** Preheat a grill or grill pan over medium-high heat. Rub the chicken breast with olive oil, salt, and pepper. Grill for about 6-7 minutes on each side, or until fully cooked and no longer pink in the center. Remove from the grill and let it rest for a few minutes before slicing.
2. **Prepare the Dressing:** In a small bowl, whisk together olive oil, orange juice, lime juice, honey (or sweetener), salt, and pepper until well combined.
3. **Assemble the Salad:** In a large bowl, combine the mixed salad greens, sliced avocado, cherry tomatoes, red onion, and cucumber. Add the sliced grilled chicken on top.
4. **Dress the Salad:** Drizzle the citrus dressing over the salad and toss gently to combine.
5. **Serve:** Enjoy immediately as a refreshing and nutritious lunch.

Nutrition Information (Per Serving)

Calories	450
Protein	30g
Carbohydrates	20g
Dietary Fiber	10g
Sugars	5g
Fat	30g
Saturated Fat	4g

"Rise above the noise."

QUICK NOTES

TIPS FOR CUSTOMIZATION

- **Add Nuts:** Sprinkle with sliced almonds or walnuts for added crunch and healthy fats.
- **Vegetable Variations:** Include other vegetables like bell peppers, radishes, or carrots for extra nutrients.
- **Protein Options:** Substitute grilled chicken with grilled shrimp, tofu, or chickpeas for a different protein source.

Why is this recipe good for PCOS?

This salad is rich in protein from the grilled chicken, which helps regulate blood sugar levels and promotes satiety. The healthy fats from avocado support hormone balance, while the variety of vegetables provides essential vitamins and minerals. The citrus dressing adds flavor without excess sugar, making this a nutritious and satisfying meal for women managing PCOS.

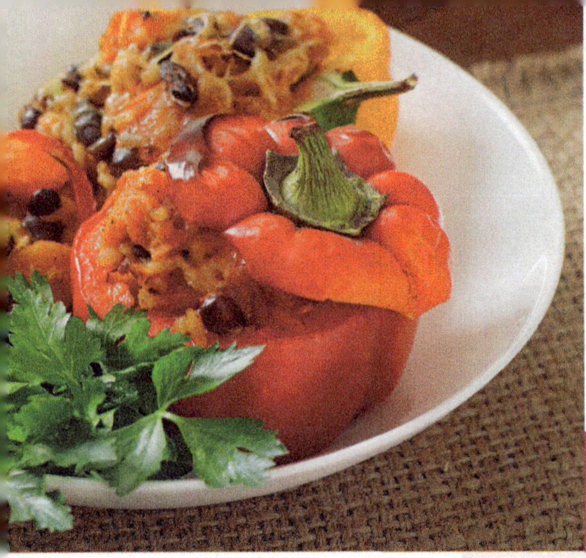

Quinoa and Black Bean Stuffed Bell Peppers

SERVING SIZE
Serves 2 (1 stuffed pepper per serving

INGREDIENTS

- 2 large bell peppers (any color)
- 1/2 cup quinoa, rinsed and drained
- 1 cup vegetable broth or water
- 1 can (15 oz) black beans, rinsed and drained
- 1 cup corn (fresh, frozen, or canned)
- 1/2 teaspoon cumin
- 1/2 teaspoon chili powder
- Salt and pepper to taste
- 1/4 cup fresh cilantro, chopped (optional)
- Juice of 1 lime
- *Optional* Avocado slices for topping

DIRECTIONS

1. **Preheat Oven:** Preheat your oven to 375°F (190°C).
2. **Cook Quinoa:** In a medium saucepan, combine quinoa and vegetable broth (or water). Bring to a boil, then reduce heat to low, cover, and simmer for about 15 minutes, or until the quinoa is fluffy and the liquid is absorbed. Remove from heat and let it sit for a few minutes.
3. **Prepare Bell Peppers:** While the quinoa is cooking, cut the tops off the bell peppers and remove the seeds and membranes. Place the peppers upright in a baking dish.
4. **Mix Filling:** In a large bowl, combine the cooked quinoa, black beans, corn, cumin, chili powder, salt, pepper, cilantro (if using), and lime juice. Mix well to combine.
5. **Stuff Peppers:** Spoon the quinoa and black bean mixture into each bell pepper, packing it down gently.
6. **Bake:** Cover the baking dish with foil and bake in the preheated oven for 25-30 minutes. Remove the foil and bake for an additional 10 minutes, or until the peppers are tender.
7. **Serve:** Remove from the oven and let cool slightly. Serve warm, topped with avocado slices if desired.

Nutrition Information (Per Serving)

Calories	350
Protein	12g
Carbohydrates	60g
Dietary Fiber	15g
Sugars	5g
Fat	6g
Saturated Fat	1g

"You are worthy of love."

QUICK NOTES

TIPS FOR CUSTOMIZATION

- **Add Cheese:** For a dairy-free option, sprinkle with nutritional yeast for a cheesy flavor.
- **Spice it Up:** Add diced jalapeños or red pepper flakes for extra heat.
- **Vegetable Variations:** Include diced zucchini, mushrooms, or spinach in the filling for added nutrition.

Why is this recipe good for PCOS?

This dish is high in fiber from quinoa and black beans, which helps regulate blood sugar levels and promotes satiety. The combination of protein and complex carbohydrates makes it a balanced meal option. Bell peppers are rich in vitamins and antioxidants, making this a nutritious and satisfying choice for women managing PCOS.

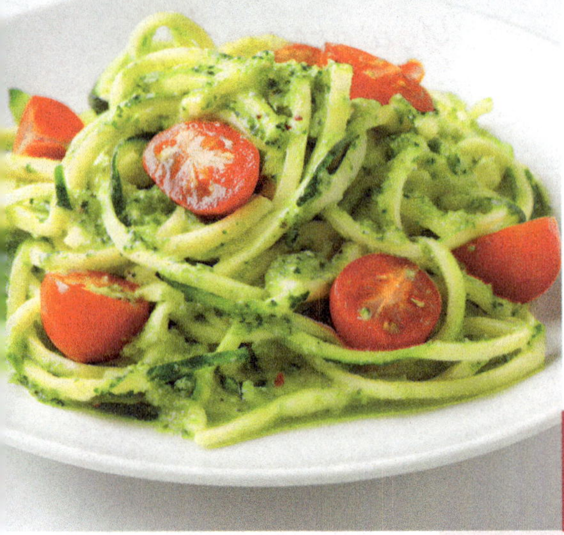

Zucchini Noodles with Pesto and Cherry Tomatoes

SERVING SIZE
Serves 1

INGREDIENTS

- 2 medium zucchinis, spiralized into noodles
- 1 cup cherry tomatoes, halved
- 1/4 cup basil pesto (store-bought or homemade)
- 1 tablespoon olive oil
- Salt and pepper to taste
- *Optional*
  Grated nutritional yeast or pine nuts for garnish
  Optional: Fresh basil leaves for garnish

DIRECTIONS

1. **Prepare Zucchini Noodles:** Spiralize the zucchinis into noodles and set aside.
2. **Sauté Cherry Tomatoes:** In a large skillet, heat olive oil over medium heat. Add the halved cherry tomatoes and sauté for about 3-4 minutes, until they start to soften.
3. **Add Zucchini Noodles:** Add the spiralized zucchini noodles to the skillet and cook for an additional 2-3 minutes, stirring gently until the noodles are tender but still slightly crisp.
4. **Mix in Pesto:** Remove the skillet from heat and stir in the basil pesto until the zucchini noodles and tomatoes are well coated.
5. **Serve:** Season with salt and pepper to taste. Serve immediately, garnished with nutritional yeast or pine nuts and fresh basil leaves if desired.

Nutrition Information (Per Serving)

Calories	250
Protein	6g
Carbohydrates	15g
Dietary Fiber	4g
Sugars	4g
Fat	20g
Saturated Fat	3g

"Courage is your superpower."

QUICK NOTES

TIPS FOR CUSTOMIZATION

- **Add Protein:** Include grilled chicken, shrimp, or tofu for an extra protein boost.
- **Vegetable Variations:** Incorporate other vegetables like bell peppers, spinach, or mushrooms for added nutrition.
- **Spice it Up:** Add red pepper flakes or a squeeze of lemon juice for extra flavor.

Why is this recipe good for PCOS?

Zucchini noodles are low in carbohydrates and calories, making them an excellent choice for managing blood sugar levels. The healthy fats from olive oil and pesto support hormone balance, while the cherry tomatoes provide antioxidants and vitamins. This dish is quick to prepare, nutrient-dense, and satisfying, making it a great option for women managing PCOS.

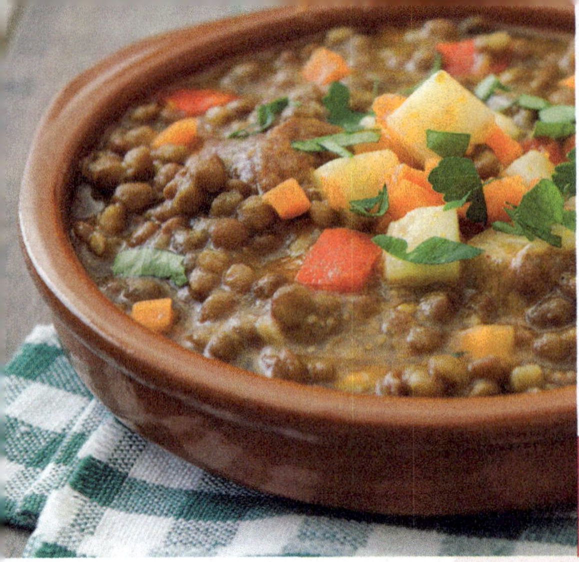

Lentil Soup with Spinach and Carrots

SERVING SIZE
Serves 4

INGREDIENTS

- 1 cup dried lentils (green or brown), rinsed and drained
- 1 tablespoon olive oil
- 1 medium onion, diced
- 2 cloves garlic, minced
- 2 medium carrots, diced
- 2 celery stalks, diced
- 4 cups vegetable broth or water
- 1 teaspoon cumin
- 1 teaspoon thyme
- Salt and pepper to taste
- 2 cups fresh spinach, chopped
- Juice of 1 lemon (optional, for serving)

DIRECTIONS

1. **Sauté Vegetables:** In a large pot, heat olive oil over medium heat. Add the diced onion, garlic, carrots, and celery. Sauté for about 5-7 minutes, or until the vegetables are softened.
2. **Add Lentils and Broth:** Stir in the rinsed lentils, vegetable broth (or water), cumin, thyme, salt, and pepper. Bring to a boil, then reduce heat to low and simmer for about 25-30 minutes, or until the lentils are tender.
3. **Add Spinach:** Once the lentils are cooked, stir in the chopped spinach and cook for an additional 2-3 minutes until wilted.
4. **Serve:** Remove from heat and adjust seasoning if needed. Serve hot, with a squeeze of lemon juice if desired.

Nutrition Information (Per Serving)

Calories	200
Protein	12g
Carbohydrates	35g
Dietary Fiber	12g
Sugars	3g
Fat	4g
Saturated Fat	1g

"Create your own path."

QUICK NOTES

TIPS FOR CUSTOMIZATION

- **Add Protein:** Include diced chicken, turkey, or tofu for an extra protein boost.
- **Spice it Up:** Add red pepper flakes or a dash of hot sauce for extra heat.
- **Vegetable Variations:** Incorporate other vegetables like zucchini, bell peppers, or kale for added nutrition.

Why is this recipe good for PCOS?

Lentils are an excellent source of plant-based protein and fiber, which help regulate blood sugar levels and promote satiety. The combination of spinach and carrots provides essential vitamins and minerals, while the healthy fats from olive oil support hormone balance. This hearty soup is low in carbohydrates and packed with nutrients, making it a comforting and nutritious option for women managing PCOS.

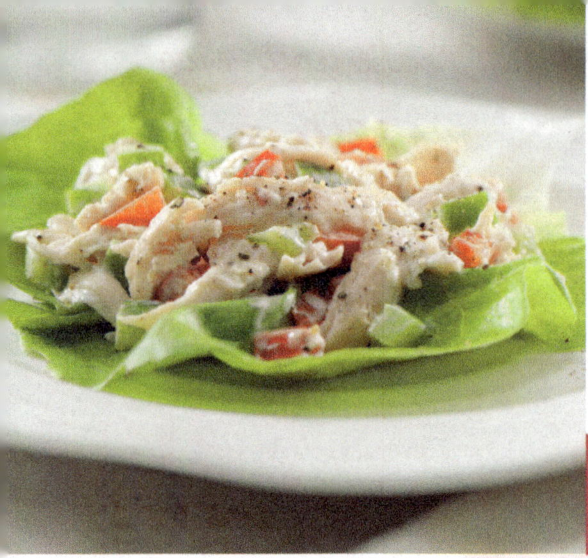

Tuna Salad Lettuce Wraps with Olive Oil Dressing

SERVING SIZE
Serves 2 (2 wraps per serving)

INGREDIENTS

- 1 can (5 oz) tuna in water, drained
- 1/4 cup celery, finely diced
- 1/4 cup red onion, finely diced
- 1/4 cup cucumber, diced
- 1 tablespoon capers (optional)
- 2 tablespoons olive oil
- 1 tablespoon lemon juice
- Salt and pepper to taste
- 4 large lettuce leaves (such as romaine or butter lettuce)
- *Optional*
  Fresh herbs (like dill or parsley) for garnish

DIRECTIONS

1. **Prepare Tuna Salad:** In a medium bow!, combine the drained tuna, diced celery, red onion, cucumber, and capers (if using).
2. **Make Dressing:** In a small bowl, whisk together the olive oil, lemon juice, salt, and pepper until well combined.
3. **Combine:** Pour the dressing over the tuna mixture and stir until everything is well coated.
4. **Assemble Wraps:** Place a generous scoop of the tuna salad onto each lettuce leaf, folding the leaf around the filling to create a wrap.
5. **Serve:** Garnish with fresh herbs if desired and serve immediately.

Nutrition Information (Per Serving)

Calories	250
Protein	30g
Carbohydrates	6g
Dietary Fiber	2g
Sugars	1g
Fat	14g
Saturated Fat	2g

"You define your success."

QUICK NOTES

TIPS FOR CUSTOMIZATION

- **Add Veggies:** Include additional vegetables like bell peppers, shredded carrots, or avocado for extra nutrition.
- **Spice it Up:** Add a dash of hot sauce or red pepper flakes for a spicy kick.
- **Protein Variations:** Substitute tuna with canned salmon or shredded chicken for variety.

Why is this recipe good for PCOS?

This tuna salad is high in protein, which helps regulate blood sugar levels and promotes satiety. The healthy fats from olive oil support hormone balance, while the fresh vegetables provide essential vitamins and minerals. Using lettuce wraps instead of bread keeps the meal low in carbohydrates, making it a nutritious and satisfying option for women managing PCOS.

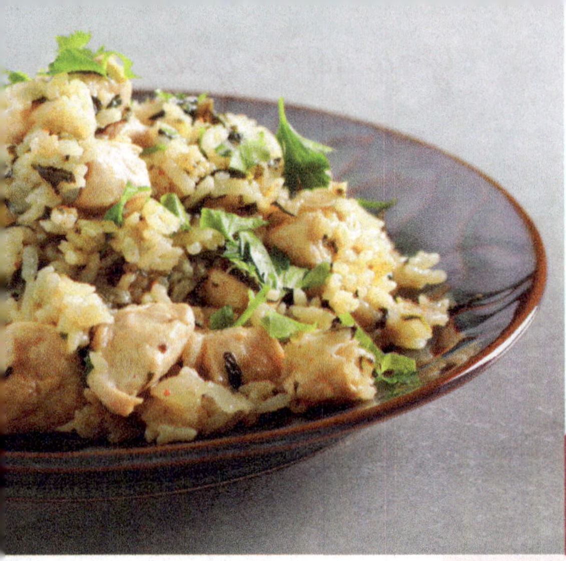

Cauliflower Fried Rice with Vegetables and Chicken

SERVING SIZE
Serves 2

INGREDIENTS

- 1 medium head of cauliflower, riced (or 4 cups pre-riced cauliflower)
- 1 cup cooked chicken breast, diced
  1 cup mixed vegetables (such as peas, carrots, and bell peppers)
- 2 tablespoons olive oil or avocado oil
- 2 cloves garlic, minced
- 2 eggs, lightly beaten
- 3 tablespoons low-sodium soy sauce or tamari (for gluten-free)
- Salt and pepper to taste
- *Optional* Green onions, sliced, for garnish
- *Optional* Sesame seeds for garnish

DIRECTIONS

1. **Prepare Cauliflower Rice:** If using a whole head of cauliflower, remove the leaves and stem, and cut it into florets. Pulse in a food processor until it resembles rice. Set aside.
2. **Sauté Vegetables:** In a large skillet or wok, heat 1 tablespoon of oil over medium heat. Add the minced garlic and sauté for about 30 seconds until fragrant. Add the mixed vegetables and cook for 3-4 minutes until tender.
3. **Add Chicken:** Stir in the diced cooked chicken and cook for an additional 2 minutes until heated through.
4. **Push to Side:** Push the vegetable and chicken mixture to one side of the skillet. Add the remaining tablespoon of oil to the empty side and pour in the beaten eggs. Scramble the eggs until fully cooked, then mix them into the vegetable and chicken mixture.
5. **Add Cauliflower Rice:** Add the riced cauliflower to the skillet and pour in the soy sauce or tamari. Stir well to combine all ingredients and cook for an additional 5-7 minutes, stirring occasionally, until the cauliflower is tender.
6. **Serve:** Season with salt and pepper to taste. Garnish with sliced green onions and sesame seeds if desired. Serve hot.

Nutrition Information (Per Serving)

Calories	350
Protein	30g
Carbohydrates	20g
Dietary Fiber	6g
Sugars	4g
Fat	18g
Saturated Fat	3g

"Be the change you seek."

QUICK NOTES

TIPS FOR CUSTOMIZATION

- **Add More Veggies:** Include additional vegetables like broccoli, zucchini, or snap peas for extra nutrition.
- **Spice it Up:** Add a dash of sriracha or red pepper flakes for a spicy kick.
- **Protein Variations:** Substitute chicken with shrimp, tofu, or tempeh for a different protein source.

Why is this recipe good for PCOS?

This cauliflower fried rice is low in carbohydrates and high in fiber, making it an excellent choice for managing blood sugar levels. The combination of protein from chicken and eggs helps promote satiety, while the variety of vegetables provides essential vitamins and minerals. This dish is nutrient-dense and satisfying, making it a great option for women managing PCOS.

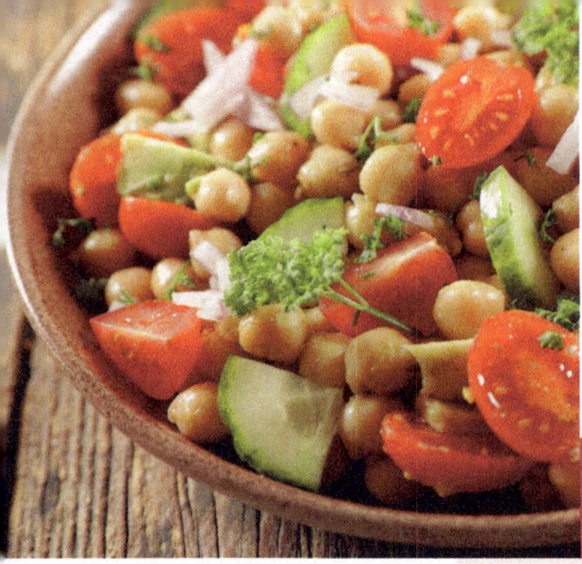

Chickpea Salad with Cucumber, Tomatoes, and Lemon Dressing

SERVING SIZE
Serves 2

INGREDIENTS

- 1 can (15 oz) chickpeas, rinsed and drained
- 1 cup cucumber, diced
- 1 cup cherry tomatoes, halved
- 1/4 cup red onion, finely diced
- 1/4 cup fresh parsley, chopped
- 2 tablespoons olive oil
- Juice of 1 lemon
- Salt and pepper to taste
- *Optional*
  Feta cheese (dairy-free if needed) for topping

DIRECTIONS

1. **Prepare Salad Ingredients:** In a large bowl, combine the rinsed chickpeas, diced cucumber, halved cherry tomatoes, diced red onion, and chopped parsley.
2. **Make Dressing:** In a small bowl, whisk together the olive oil, lemon juice, salt, and pepper until well combined.
3. **Combine:** Pour the dressing over the salad and toss gently to combine all ingredients.
4. **Serve:** If desired, top with feta cheese before serving. Enjoy immediately or refrigerate for 30 minutes to allow the flavors to meld.

Nutrition Information (Per Serving)

Calories	250
Protein	10g
Carbohydrates	30g
Dietary Fiber	8g
Sugars	4g
Fat	12g
Saturated Fat	2g

"Your potential is limitless."

QUICK NOTES

TIPS FOR CUSTOMIZATION

- **Add Veggies:** Include additional vegetables like bell peppers, radishes, or avocado for extra nutrition.
- **Spice it Up:** Add a pinch of cumin or paprika for added flavor.
- **Protein Variations:** Substitute chickpeas with black beans or kidney beans for variety.

Why is this recipe good for PCOS?

Chickpeas are a great source of plant-based protein and fiber, which help regulate blood sugar levels and promote satiety. The fresh vegetables provide essential vitamins and minerals, while the healthy fats from olive oil support hormone balance. This salad is low in refined sugars and high in nutrients, making it a nutritious and satisfying option for women managing PCOS.

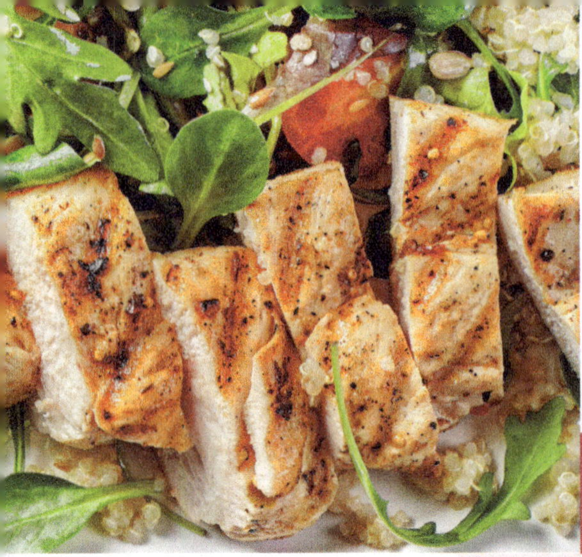

Turkey and Vegetable Skillet with Quinoa

SERVING SIZE
Serves 4

INGREDIENTS

- 1 pound ground turkey (lean)
- 1 cup quinoa, rinsed and drained
- 2 cups vegetable broth or water
- 1 tablespoon olive oil
- 1 medium onion, diced
- 2 cloves garlic, minced
- 1 cup bell peppers, diced (any color)
- 1 cup zucchini, diced
- 1 cup spinach, chopped
- 1 teaspoon Italian seasoning
- Salt and pepper to taste
- *Optional* Fresh parsley for garnish

DIRECTIONS

1. **Cook Quinoa:** In a medium saucepan, combine quinoa and vegetable broth (or water). Bring to a boil, then reduce heat to low, cover, and simmer for about 15 minutes, or until the quinoa is fluffy and the liquid is absorbed. Remove from heat and set aside.
2. **Sauté Vegetables:** In a large skillet, heat olive oil over medium heat. Add the diced onion and garlic, and sauté for about 3-4 minutes until the onion is translucent.
3. **Add Turkey:** Add the ground turkey to the skillet, breaking it apart with a spoon. Cook until browned and fully cooked, about 5-7 minutes.
4. **Add Vegetables:** Stir in the diced bell peppers, zucchini, and Italian seasoning. Cook for an additional 5-7 minutes until the vegetables are tender.
5. **Combine with Quinoa:** Add the cooked quinoa and chopped spinach to the skillet. Stir well to combine and cook for another 2-3 minutes until the spinach is wilted.
6. **Serve:** Season with salt and pepper to taste. Garnish with fresh parsley if desired. Serve warm.

Nutrition Information (Per Serving)

Calories	350
Protein	30g
Carbohydrates	35g
Dietary Fiber	6g
Sugars	3g
Fat	10g
Saturated Fat	2g

"Trust your instincts."

QUICK NOTES

TIPS FOR CUSTOMIZATION

- **Add More Veggies:** Include additional vegetables like carrots, broccoli, or peas for extra nutrition.
- **Spice it Up:** Add red pepper flakes or hot sauce for a spicy kick.
- **Protein Variations:** Substitute ground turkey with ground chicken, beef, or plant-based meat alternatives for variety.

Why is this recipe good for PCOS?

This skillet dish is high in protein from the ground turkey and quinoa, which helps regulate blood sugar levels and promotes satiety. The variety of vegetables provides essential vitamins and minerals, while the healthy fats from olive oil support hormone balance. This one-pan meal is nutrient-dense and satisfying, making it a great option for women managing PCOS.

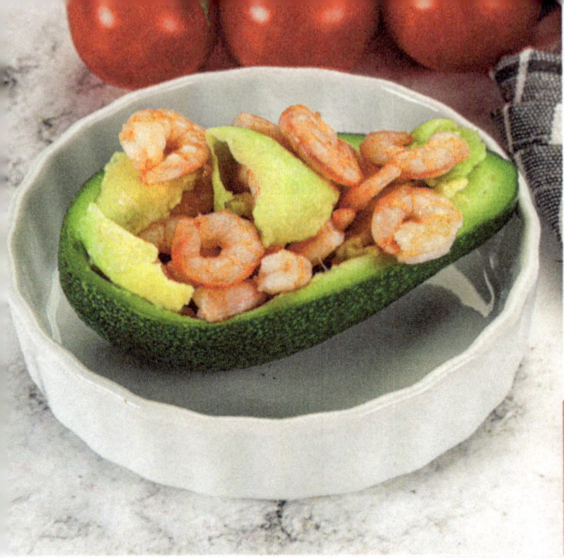

Stuffed Avocado with Shrimp and Mango Salsa

SERVING SIZE
Serves 2 (1 stuffed avocado half per serving)

INGREDIENTS

- 2 ripe avocados, halved and pitted
- 1 cup cooked shrimp, peeled and deveined
- 1 cup mango, diced
- 1/2 cup red bell pepper, diced
- 1/4 cup red onion, finely diced
- 1/4 cup fresh cilantro, chopped
- Juice of 1 lime
- Salt and pepper to taste

DIRECTIONS

1. **Prepare Mango Salsa:** In a medium bowl, combine the diced mango, red bell pepper, red onion, cilantro, lime juice, salt, and pepper. Mix well and set aside to allow the flavors to meld.
2. **Stuff Avocados:** Take the halved avocados and scoop out a small portion of the flesh to create a larger cavity for the filling. You can chop the scooped-out avocado and mix it into the shrimp and mango salsa if desired.
3. **Combine Shrimp and Salsa:** Gently fold the cooked shrimp into the mango salsa mixture.
4. **Fill Avocados:** Spoon the shrimp and mango salsa mixture into each avocado half, filling them generously.
5. **Serve:** Enjoy immediately as a refreshing and nutritious lunch or snack.

Nutrition Information (Per Serving)

Calories	350
Protein	20g
Carbohydrates	30g
Dietary Fiber	12g
Sugars	5g
Fat	22g
Saturated Fat	3g

"You are a force of nature."

QUICK NOTES

TIPS FOR CUSTOMIZATION

- **Add Heat:** Include diced jalapeños or a dash of hot sauce for a spicy kick.
- **Protein Variations:** Substitute shrimp with cooked chicken, crab, or tofu for variety.
- **Extra Flavor:** Drizzle with additional lime juice or a sprinkle of chili powder for added flavor.

Why is this recipe good for PCOS?

This dish is rich in healthy fats from avocados, which help regulate blood sugar levels and promote satiety. The shrimp provides high-quality protein, while the mango and vegetables add essential vitamins, minerals, and antioxidants. This recipe is low in carbohydrates and nutrient-dense, making it a delicious and satisfying option for women managing PCOS.

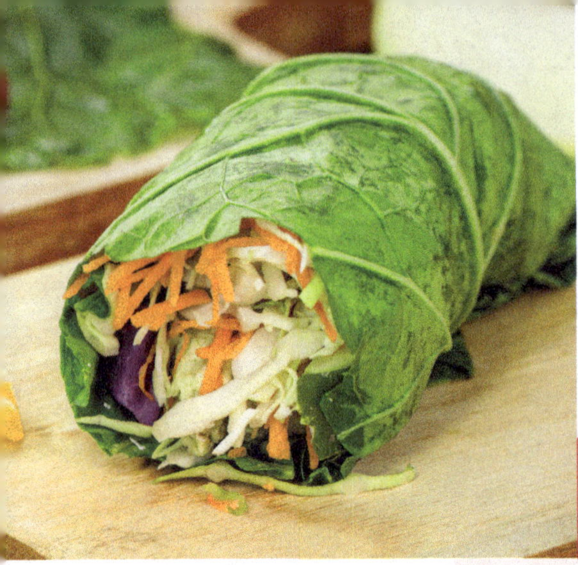

Roasted Vegetable and Hummus Wrap in Collard Greens

SERVING SIZE
Serves 2 (2 wraps per serving)

INGREDIENTS

- 4 large collard green leaves, stems removed
- 1 cup mixed vegetables (such as bell peppers, zucchini, and carrots), diced
- 1 tablespoon olive oil
- Salt and pepper to taste
- 1/2 teaspoon garlic powder (optional)
- 1/2 cup hummus (store-bought or homemade)
- *Optional* Fresh herbs (like parsley or cilantro) for garnish

DIRECTIONS

1. **Preheat Oven:** Preheat your oven to 400°F (200°C).
2. **Roast Vegetables:** On a baking sheet, toss the diced mixed vegetables with olive oil, salt, pepper, and garlic powder (if using). Spread them out in a single layer and roast in the preheated oven for about 20-25 minutes, or until tender and slightly caramelized.
3. **Prepare Collard Greens:** While the vegetables are roasting, prepare the collard green leaves. Blanch them in boiling water for about 30 seconds to soften, then transfer to an ice bath to cool. Pat dry with a paper towel.
4. **Assemble Wraps:** Spread a generous layer of hummus on each collard green leaf. Top with the roasted vegetables and sprinkle with fresh herbs if desired.
5. **Wrap:** Roll the collard greens tightly, starting from the stem end, and tuck in the sides as you go to create a wrap.
6. **Serve:** Cut the wraps in half and serve immediately, or wrap in parchment paper for a portable meal.

Nutrition Information (Per Serving)

Calories	300
Protein	10g
Carbohydrates	30g
Dietary Fiber	10g
Sugars	5g
Fat	18g
Saturated Fat	2g

"Celebrate your uniqueness."

QUICK NOTES

TIPS FOR CUSTOMIZATION

- **Add Protein:** Include cooked chickpeas, grilled chicken, or tofu for an extra protein boost.
- **Vegetable Variations:** Use any seasonal vegetables or your favorites for roasting.
- **Spice it Up:** Add a sprinkle of red pepper flakes or a drizzle of hot sauce for extra heat.

Why is this recipe good for PCOS?

This wrap is low in carbohydrates and high in fiber, making it an excellent choice for managing blood sugar levels. The healthy fats from olive oil and hummus support hormone balance, while the variety of roasted vegetables provides essential vitamins and minerals. Using collard greens instead of traditional wraps keeps the meal nutrient-dense and satisfying, making it a great option for women managing PCOS.

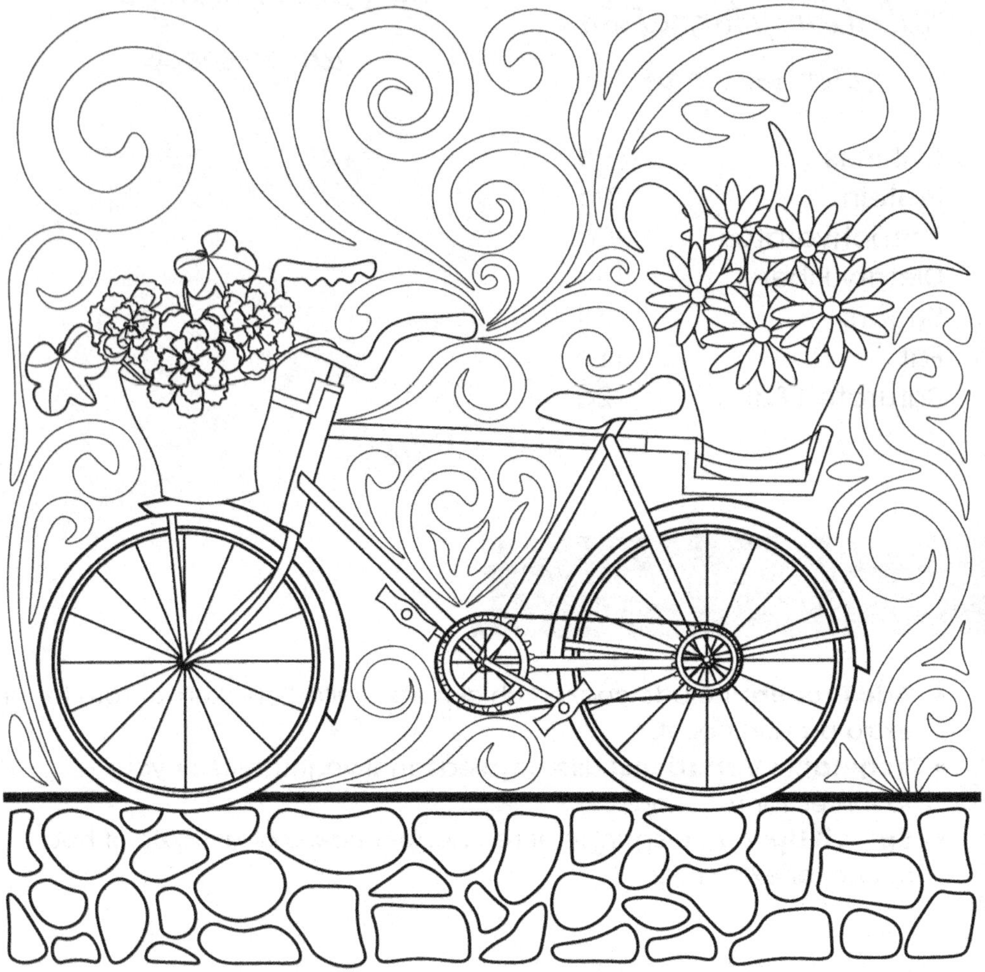

so, one of the amazing bonding times that John and myself enjoy a lot is, yeah, biking... or cycling... My husband's a bit of a pro when he was younger and I got to embrace that outdoor freedom (+workout) of riding a bike when we got married. We own pretty standard mountain bikes but we're really huge Tour de France fans :).

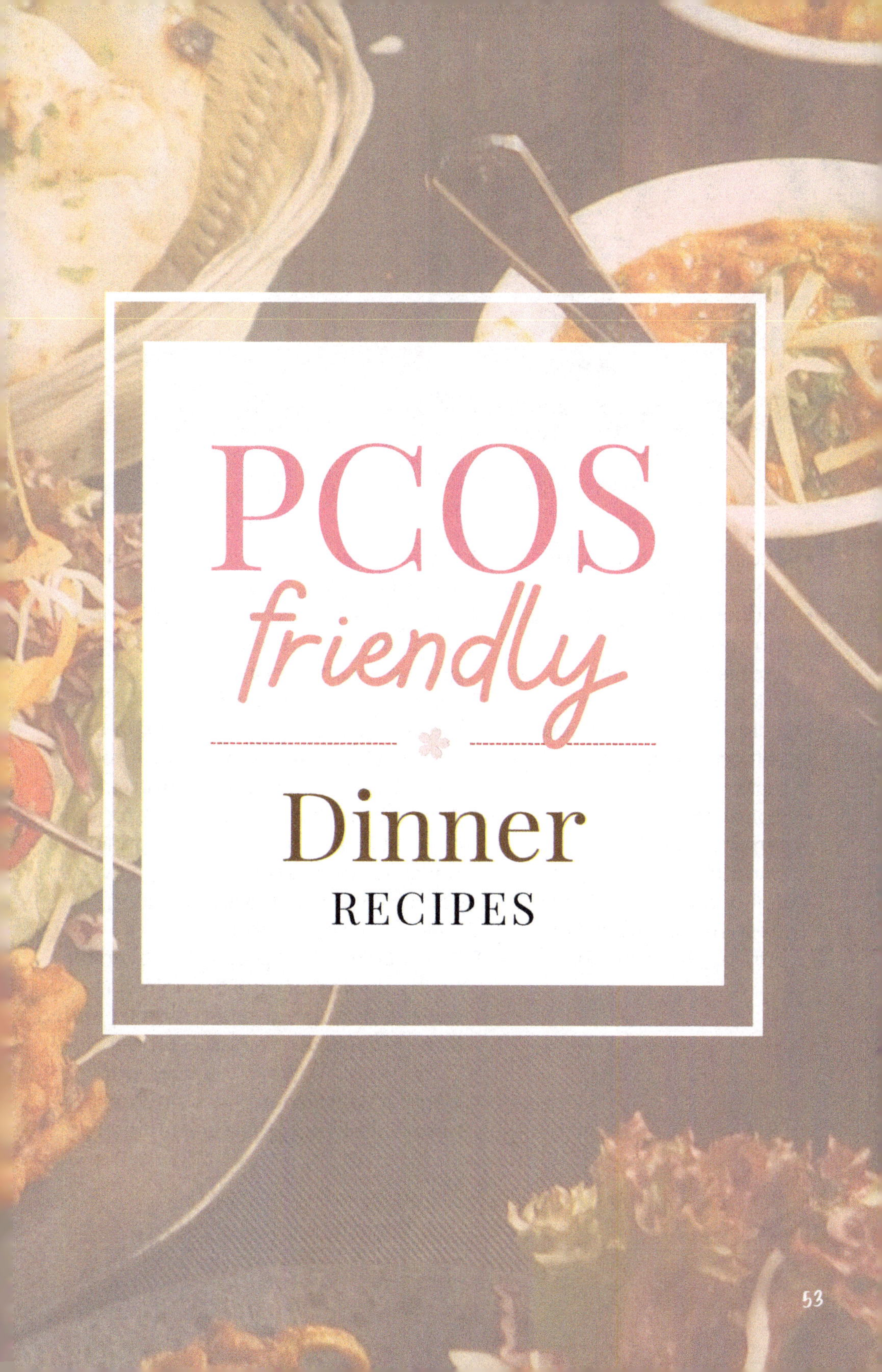

PCOS friendly

Dinner RECIPES

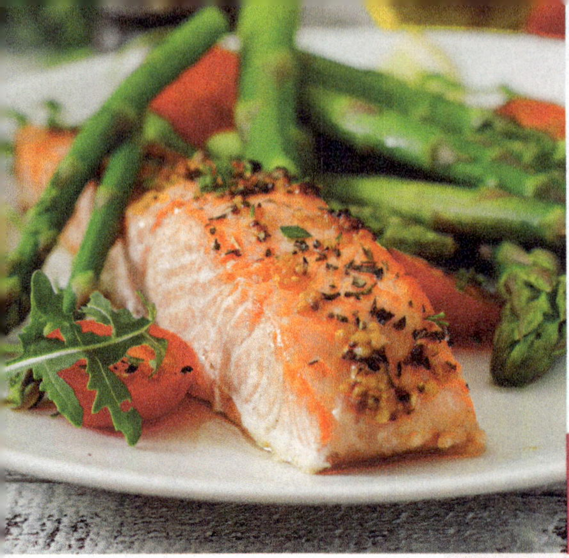

Baked Salmon with Asparagus and Lemon

SERVING SIZE
Serves 2

INGREDIENTS

- 2 salmon fillets (about 6 ounces each)
- 1 bunch asparagus, trimmed
- 2 tablespoons olive oil
- Juice of 1 lemon
- 2 cloves garlic, minced
- Salt and pepper to taste
- *Optional* Lemon slices for garnish
- *Optional* Fresh herbs (like dill or parsley) for garnish

DIRECTIONS

1. **Preheat Oven:** Preheat your oven to 400°F (200°C).
2. **Prepare Baking Sheet:** Line a baking sheet with parchment paper or lightly grease it with cooking spray.
3. **Arrange Salmon and Asparagus:** Place the salmon fillets in the center of the baking sheet. Arrange the trimmed asparagus around the salmon.
4. **Season:** In a small bowl, whisk together olive oil, lemon juice, minced garlic, salt, and pepper. Drizzle the mixture over the salmon and asparagus, ensuring everything is well coated.
5. **Bake:** Bake in the preheated oven for 12-15 minutes, or until the salmon is cooked through and flakes easily with a fork, and the asparagus is tender.
6. **Serve:** Remove from the oven and garnish with lemon slices and fresh herbs if desired. Serve immediately.

Nutrition Information (Per Serving)

Calories	350
Protein	30g
Carbohydrates	8g
Dietary Fiber	4g
Sugars	2g
Fat	22g
Saturated Fat	4g

"Keep pushing forward."

QUICK NOTES

TIPS FOR CUSTOMIZATION

- **Add Vegetables:** Include other vegetables like cherry tomatoes or bell peppers for added nutrition.
- **Spice it Up:** Sprinkle with red pepper flakes or your favorite seasoning blend for extra flavor.
- **Protein Variations:** Substitute salmon with other fish like trout or cod, or use chicken breast for a different protein source.

Why is this recipe good for PCOS?

Baked salmon is rich in omega-3 fatty acids, which help reduce inflammation and support hormone balance. Asparagus is low in carbohydrates and high in fiber, making it an excellent choice for managing blood sugar levels. This dish is nutrient-dense, easy to prepare, and provides a satisfying meal for women managing PCOS.

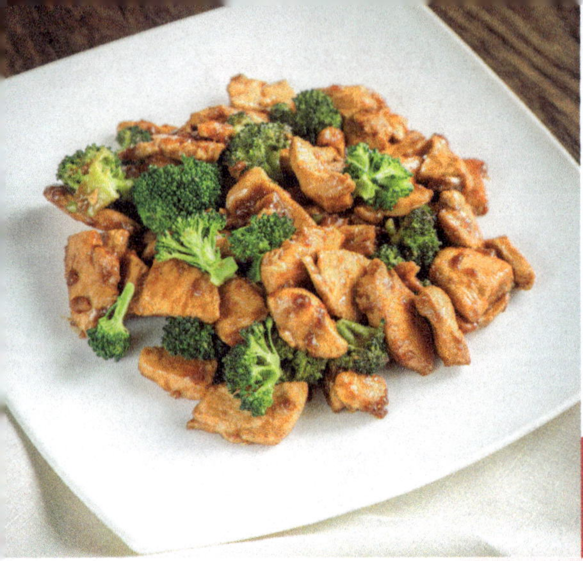

Stir-Fried Tofu with Broccoli and Brown Rice

SERVING SIZE
Serves 2

INGREDIENTS

- 1 block (14 oz) firm tofu, drained and pressed
- 2 cups broccoli florets
- 1 cup cooked brown rice
- 2 tablespoons olive oil or sesame oil
- 2 cloves garlic, minced
- 1 tablespoon fresh ginger, minced
- 3 tablespoons low-sodium soy sauce or tamari (for gluten-free)
- 1 tablespoon rice vinegar
- Salt and pepper to taste
- *Optional* Sesame seeds for garnish
- *Optional* Green onions, sliced, for garnish

DIRECTIONS

1. **Prepare Tofu:** Cut the pressed tofu into bite-sized cubes.
2. **Cook Tofu:** In a large skillet or wok, heat 1 tablespoon of oil over medium-high heat. Add the tofu cubes and cook until golden brown on all sides, about 5-7 minutes. Remove the tofu from the skillet and set aside.
3. **Sauté Vegetables:** In the same skillet, add the remaining tablespoon of oil. Add the minced garlic and ginger, and sauté for about 30 seconds until fragrant. Add the broccoli florets and stir-fry for about 3-4 minutes, or until tender-crisp.
4. **Combine Ingredients:** Return the cooked tofu to the skillet. Add the cooked brown rice, soy sauce, and rice vinegar. Stir well to combine and cook for an additional 2-3 minutes until everything is heated through.
5. **Serve:** Season with salt and pepper to taste. Garnish with sesame seeds and sliced green onions if desired. Serve warm.

Nutrition Information (Per Serving)

Calories	400
Protein	20g
Carbohydrates	50g
Dietary Fiber	8g
Sugars	2g
Fat	15g
Saturated Fat	2g

"You are a warrior."

QUICK NOTES

TIPS FOR CUSTOMIZATION

- **Add More Veggies:** Include other vegetables like bell peppers, snap peas, or carrots for added nutrition.
- **Spice it Up:** Add red pepper flakes or a dash of hot sauce for extra heat.
- **Protein Variations:** Substitute tofu with tempeh or chicken for a different protein source.

Why is this recipe good for PCOS?

This stir-fry is rich in plant-based protein from tofu, which helps regulate blood sugar levels and promotes satiety. Broccoli is high in fiber and low in carbohydrates, making it an excellent choice for managing PCOS. The combination of healthy fats from olive oil and whole grains from brown rice provides a balanced meal that is both nutritious and satisfying.

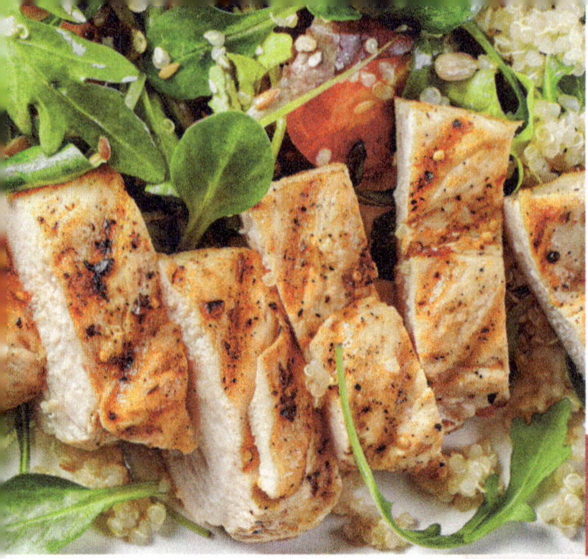

Turkey and Vegetable Skillet with Quinoa

SERVING SIZE
Serves 4

INGREDIENTS

- 1 pound ground turkey (lean)
- 1 cup quinoa, rinsed and drained
- 2 cups vegetable broth or water
- 1 tablespoon olive oil
- 1 medium onion, diced
- 2 cloves garlic, minced
- 1 cup bell peppers, diced (any color)
- 1 cup zucchini, diced
- 1 cup spinach, chopped
- 1 teaspoon Italian seasoning
- Salt and pepper to taste
- *Optional* Fresh parsley for garnish

DIRECTIONS

1. **Cook Quinoa:** In a medium saucepan, combine quinoa and vegetable broth (or water). Bring to a boil, then reduce heat to low, cover, and simmer for about 15 minutes, or until the quinoa is fluffy and the liquid is absorbed. Remove from heat and set aside.
2. **Sauté Vegetables:** In a large skillet, heat olive oil over medium heat. Add the diced onion and garlic, and sauté for about 3-4 minutes until the onion is translucent.
3. **Add Turkey:** Add the ground turkey to the skillet, breaking it apart with a spoon. Cook until browned and fully cooked, about 5-7 minutes.
4. **Add Vegetables:** Stir in the diced bell peppers, zucchini, and Italian seasoning. Cook for an additional 5-7 minutes until the vegetables are tender.
5. **Combine with Quinoa:** Add the cooked quinoa and chopped spinach to the skillet. Stir well to combine and cook for another 2-3 minutes until the spinach is wilted.
6. **Serve:** Season with salt and pepper to taste. Garnish with fresh parsley if desired. Serve warm.

Nutrition Information (Per Serving)

Calories	350
Protein	30g
Carbohydrates	35g
Dietary Fiber	6g
Sugars	3g
Fat	10g
Saturated Fat	2g

"Your dreams are valid."

QUICK NOTES

TIPS FOR CUSTOMIZATION

- **Add More Veggies:** Include additional vegetables like carrots, broccoli, or peas for extra nutrition.
- **Spice it Up:** Add red pepper flakes or hot sauce for a spicy kick.
- **Protein Variations:** Substitute ground turkey with ground chicken, beef, or plant-based meat alternatives for variety.

Why is this recipe good for PCOS?

This skillet dish is high in protein from the ground turkey and quinoa, which helps regulate blood sugar levels and promotes satiety. The variety of vegetables provides essential vitamins and minerals, while the healthy fats from olive oil support hormone balance. This one-pan meal is nutrient-dense and satisfying, making it a great option for women managing PCOS.

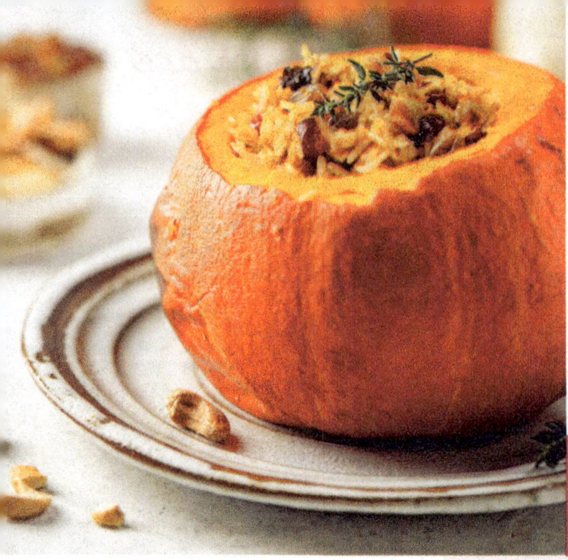

Stuffed Acorn Squash with Wild Rice and Cranberries

SERVING SIZE
Serves 4

INGREDIENTS

- 2 acorn squashes, halved and seeds removed
- 1 cup wild rice, rinsed
- 2 cups vegetable broth or water
- 1/2 cup dried cranberries (unsweetened if possible)
- 1/2 cup walnuts, chopped
- 1 small onion, diced
- 2 cloves garlic, minced
- 1 teaspoon dried thyme
- 1 teaspoon dried sage
- Salt and pepper to taste
- 2 tablespoons olive oil
- Optional Fresh parsley for garnish

DIRECTIONS

1. **Preheat Oven:** Preheat your oven to 400°F (200°C).
2. **Prepare Acorn Squash:** Place the acorn squash halves cut-side up on a baking sheet. Drizzle with 1 tablespoon of olive oil and season with salt and pepper. Roast in the preheated oven for about 30-35 minutes, or until tender.
3. **Cook Wild Rice:** In a medium saucepan, combine wild rice and vegetable broth (or water). Bring to a boil, then reduce heat to low, cover, and simmer for about 45-50 minutes, or until the rice is tender and the liquid is absorbed. Remove from heat and set aside.
4. **Sauté Vegetables:** In a skillet, heat the remaining tablespoon of olive oil over medium heat. Add the diced onion and garlic, and sauté for about 3-4 minutes until the onion is translucent.
5. **Combine Filling:** In a large bowl, combine the cooked wild rice, sautéed onion and garlic, dried cranberries, chopped walnuts, thyme, sage, salt, and pepper. Mix well to combine.
6. **Stuff Squash**: Once the acorn squash is roasted, remove it from the oven and carefully fill each half with the wild rice mixture, pressing down gently to pack it in.
7. **Bake Again:** Return the stuffed squash to the oven and bake for an additional 10-15 minutes to heat through.
8. **Serve:** Remove from the oven and garnish with fresh parsley if desired. Serve warm.

Nutrition Information (Per Serving)

Calories	350
Protein	10g
Carbohydrates	60g
Dietary Fiber	10g
Sugars	8g
Fat	12g
Saturated Fat	2g

"Stay fierce and fearless."

QUICK NOTES

TIPS FOR CUSTOMIZATION

- **Add Protein:** Include cooked chicken, turkey, or plant-based protein for an extra protein boost.
- **Vegetable Variations:** Incorporate other vegetables like spinach, mushrooms, or bell peppers into the filling.
- **Spice it Up:** Add a pinch of cayenne pepper or red pepper flakes for a spicy kick.

Why is this recipe good for PCOS?

This stuffed acorn squash is rich in fiber from wild rice and vegetables, which helps regulate blood sugar levels and promotes satiety. The healthy fats from walnuts support hormone balance, while the cranberries provide antioxidants. This dish is nutrient-dense, delicious, and perfect for a comforting meal for women managing PCOS.

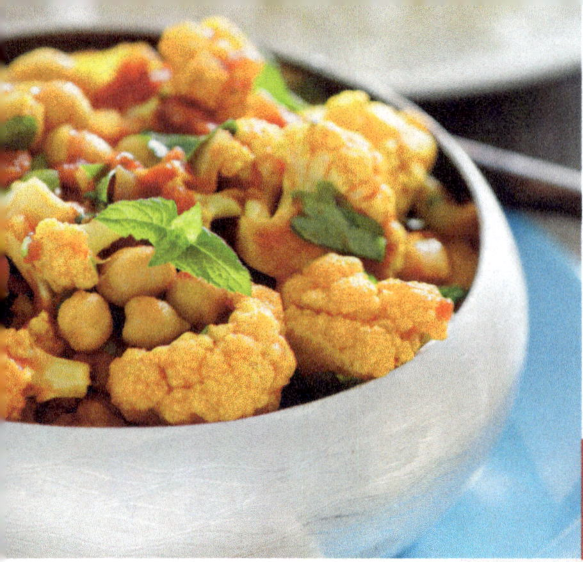

Cauliflower Curry with Chickpeas and Spinach

SERVING SIZE
Serves 4

INGREDIENTS

- 1 medium head of cauliflower, cut into florets
- 1 can (15 oz) chickpeas, rinsed and drained
- 2 cups fresh spinach, chopped
- 1 medium onion, diced
- 2 cloves garlic, minced
- 1 tablespoon fresh ginger, minced
- 1 can (14 oz) coconut milk (full-fat or light)
- 2 tablespoons curry powder
- 1 teaspoon cumin
- 1 tablespoon olive oil
- Salt and pepper to taste
- *Optional* Fresh cilantro for garnish
- *Optional* Cooked brown rice or quinoa for serving

DIRECTIONS

1. **Sauté Aromatics:** In a large pot or skillet, heat olive oil over medium heat. Add the diced onion, garlic, and ginger, and sauté for about 3-4 minutes until the onion is translucent.
2. **Add Spices:** Stir in the curry powder and cumin, cooking for an additional 1-2 minutes until fragrant.
3. **Add Cauliflower and Chickpeas:** Add the cauliflower florets and chickpeas to the pot, stirring to coat them with the spices.
4. **Add Coconut Milk:** Pour in the coconut milk and bring the mixture to a simmer. Reduce heat to low, cover, and cook for about 15-20 minutes, or until the cauliflower is tender.
5. **Add Spinach:** Stir in the chopped spinach and cook for an additional 2-3 minutes until wilted. Season with salt and pepper to taste.
6. **Serve:** Serve the curry warm, garnished with fresh cilantro if desired. Pair with cooked brown rice or quinoa for a complete meal.

Nutrition Information (Per Serving)

Calories	350
Protein	10g
Carbohydrates	40g
Dietary Fiber	10g
Sugars	4g
Fat	18g
Saturated Fat	12g

"You can do hard things."

QUICK NOTES

TIPS FOR CUSTOMIZATION

- **Add More Veggies:** Include other vegetables like bell peppers, peas, or carrots for added nutrition.
- **Spice it Up:** Add red pepper flakes or diced jalapeños for extra heat.
- **Protein Variations:** Substitute chickpeas with lentils or add cooked chicken or tofu for a different protein source.

Why is this recipe good for PCOS?

This cauliflower curry is rich in fiber from chickpeas and vegetables, which helps regulate blood sugar levels and promotes satiety. The healthy fats from coconut milk support hormone balance, while the spices provide anti-inflammatory benefits. This dish is nutrient-dense, flavorful, and perfect for a comforting meal for women managing PCOS.

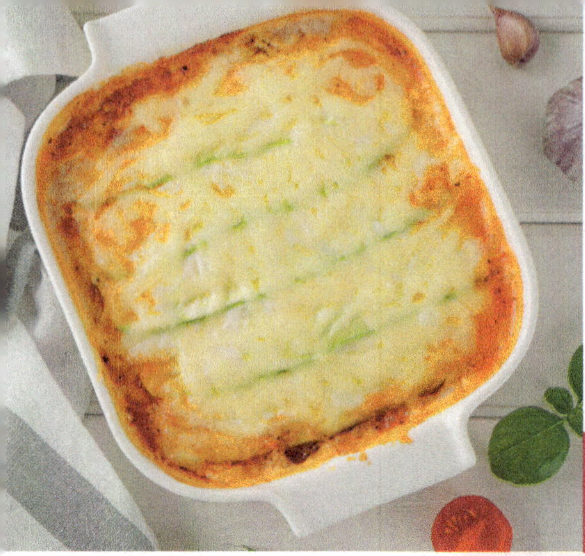

Zucchini Lasagna with Ground Turkey and Marinara

SERVING SIZE
Serves 4

INGREDIENTS

- 2 large zucchinis, sliced lengthwise into thin strips
- 1 pound ground turkey (lean)
- 2 cups marinara sauce (sugar-free if possible)
- 1 cup ricotta cheese (dairy-free if needed)
- 1 cup spinach, chopped
- 1 teaspoon Italian seasoning
- 1 teaspoon garlic powder
- Salt and pepper to taste
- 1 tablespoon olive oil
- Optional Nutritional yeast or dairy-free cheese for topping
- Optional Fresh basil for garnish

DIRECTIONS

1. **Preheat Oven:** Preheat your oven to 375°F (190°C).
2. **Prepare Zucchini:** Slice the zucchinis lengthwise into thin strips. Lay them out on paper towels and sprinkle with salt. Let them sit for about 15 minutes to draw out excess moisture, then pat dry.
3. **Cook Ground Turkey:** In a large skillet, heat olive oil over medium heat. Add the ground turkey, garlic powder, Italian seasoning, salt, and pepper. Cook until the turkey is browned and fully cooked, about 5-7 minutes. Stir in the marinara sauce and chopped spinach, and cook for an additional 2-3 minutes until the spinach is wilted.
4. **Assemble Lasagna:** In a baking dish, spread a thin layer of the turkey and marinara mixture on the bottom. Layer zucchini strips over the sauce, followed by a layer of ricotta cheese. Repeat the layers until all ingredients are used, finishing with a layer of the turkey and marinara mixture on top. If desired, sprinkle with nutritional yeast or dairy-free cheese.
5. **Bake:** Cover the baking dish with foil and bake in the preheated oven for 25-30 minutes. Remove the foil and bake for an additional 10-15 minutes, or until the top is bubbly and golden.
6. **Serve:** Remove from the oven and let it cool for a few minutes. Garnish with fresh basil if desired. Serve warm.

Nutrition Information (Per Serving)

Calories	300
Protein	25g
Carbohydrates	15g
Dietary Fiber	4g
Sugars	5g
Fat	15g
Saturated Fat	4g

"Radiate positivity."

QUICK NOTES

TIPS FOR CUSTOMIZATION

- **Add More Veggies:** Include other vegetables like mushrooms, bell peppers, or spinach in the layers for added nutrition.
- **Spice it Up:** Add red pepper flakes or Italian sausage for extra flavor.
- **Cheese Variations:** Substitute ricotta with cottage cheese or a dairy-free alternative for a different texture.

Why is this recipe good for PCOS?

This zucchini lasagna is low in carbohydrates and high in protein, making it an excellent choice for managing blood sugar levels. The zucchini provides fiber and essential nutrients, while the ground turkey offers lean protein. This dish is nutrient-dense, satisfying, and a great alternative to traditional lasagna for women managing PCOS.

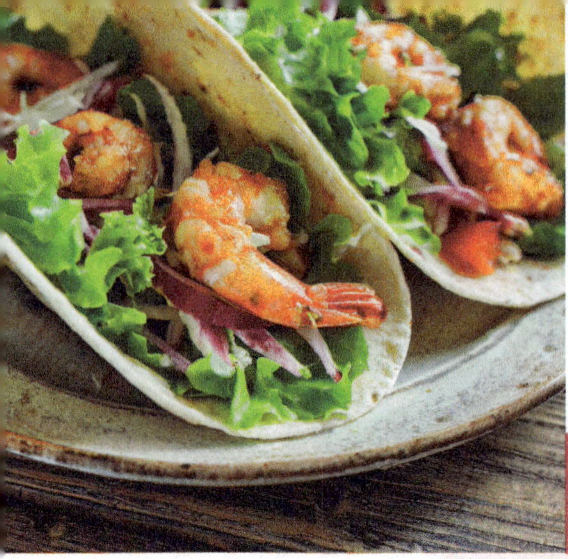

Grilled Shrimp Tacos with Cabbage Slaw

SERVING SIZE
Serves 4 (2 tacos per serving)

INGREDIENTS

- 1 pound shrimp, peeled and deveined
- 1 tablespoon olive oil
- 1 teaspoon chili powder
- 1 teaspoon cumin
- 1/2 teaspoon garlic powder
- Salt and pepper to taste
- 8 small corn tortillas (or lettuce wraps for a low-carb option)

For the Cabbage Slaw

- 2 cups green cabbage, thinly sliced
- 1 cup red cabbage, thinly sliced
- 1/2 cup carrots, grated
- 1/4 cup fresh cilantro, chopped
- Juice of 1 lime
- 1 tablespoon olive oil
- Salt and pepper to taste

DIRECTIONS

1. **Marinate Shrimp:** In a bowl, combine the shrimp, olive oil, chili powder, cumin, garlic powder, salt, and pepper. Toss to coat the shrimp evenly and let marinate for about 15-20 minutes.
2. **Prepare Cabbage Slaw:** In a separate bowl, mix together the green cabbage, red cabbage, grated carrots, cilantro, lime juice, olive oil, salt, and pepper. Toss well to combine and set aside.
3. **Grill Shrimp:** Preheat a grill or grill pan over medium-high heat. Grill the marinated shrimp for about 2-3 minutes on each side, or until they are pink and cooked through.
4. **Assemble Tacos:** Warm the corn tortillas on the grill for about 30 seconds on each side. Place a few grilled shrimp on each tortilla and top with the cabbage slaw.
5. **Serve:** Serve the tacos immediately, garnished with additional lime wedges and cilantro if desired.

Nutrition Information (Per Serving)

Calories	300
Protein	25g
Carbohydrates	30g
Dietary Fiber	6g
Sugars	3g
Fat	10g
Saturated Fat	1g

"You are a masterpiece."

QUICK NOTES

TIPS FOR CUSTOMIZATION

- **Add Heat:** Include sliced jalapeños or a drizzle of hot sauce for extra spice.
- **Vegetable Variations:** Add diced avocado or sliced radishes for additional flavor and nutrition.
- **Protein Variations:** Substitute shrimp with grilled chicken, fish, or tofu for a different protein source.

Why is this recipe good for PCOS?

These grilled shrimp tacos are high in protein, which helps regulate blood sugar levels and promotes satiety. The cabbage slaw adds fiber and essential nutrients while being low in carbohydrates. This dish is fresh, flavorful, and a great option for women managing PCOS, providing a satisfying meal without excess calories.

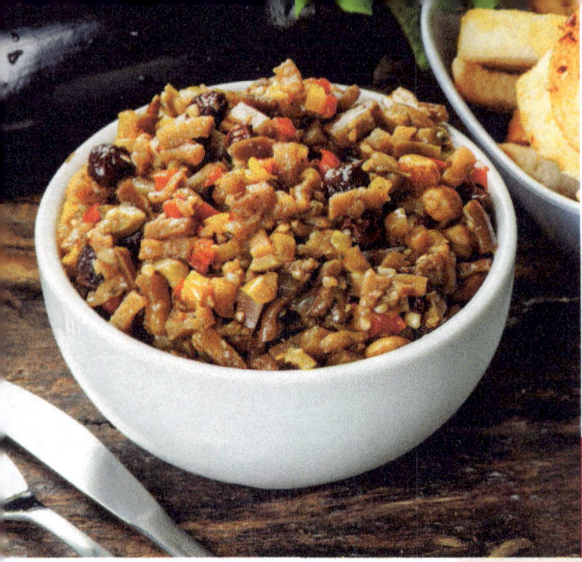

Eggplant and Chickpea Stew with Spices

SERVING SIZE
Serves 4

INGREDIENTS

- 1 medium eggplant, diced
- 1 can (15 oz) chickpeas, rinsed and drained
- 1 medium onion, diced
- 2 cloves garlic, minced
- 1 can (14 oz) diced tomatoes (with juices)
- 1 cup vegetable broth
- 1 tablespoon olive oil
- 1 teaspoon cumin
- 1 teaspoon coriander
- 1/2 teaspoon smoked paprika
- 1/2 teaspoon turmeric
- Salt and pepper to taste
- 2 cups spinach, chopped
- *Optional* Fresh cilantro for garnish
- *Optional* Lemon wedges for serving

DIRECTIONS

1. **Sauté Aromatics:** In a large pot, heat olive oil over medium heat. Add the diced onion and garlic, and sauté for about 3-4 minutes until the onion is translucent.
2. **Add Spices:** Stir in the cumin, coriander, smoked paprika, turmeric, salt, and pepper. Cook for an additional 1-2 minutes until fragrant.
3. **Add Eggplant:** Add the diced eggplant to the pot and cook for about 5-7 minutes, stirring occasionally, until the eggplant begins to soften.
4. **Add Chickpeas and Tomatoes:** Stir in the chickpeas, diced tomatoes (with juices), and vegetable broth. Bring the mixture to a simmer, then reduce heat to low and cover. Cook for about 20-25 minutes, stirring occasionally, until the eggplant is tender.
5. **Add Spinach:** Stir in the chopped spinach and cook for an additional 2-3 minutes until wilted.
6. **Serve:** Remove from heat and garnish with fresh cilantro if desired. Serve warm with lemon wedges on the side.

Nutrition Information (Per Serving)

Calories	250
Protein	10g
Carbohydrates	35g
Dietary Fiber	10g
Sugars	5g
Fat	10g
Saturated Fat	1g

"Challenge the status quo."

QUICK NOTES

TIPS FOR CUSTOMIZATION

- **Add More Veggies:** Include other vegetables like zucchini, bell peppers, or carrots for added nutrition.
- **Spice it Up:** Add red pepper flakes or diced jalapeños for extra heat.
- **Protein Variations:** Substitute chickpeas with lentils or add cooked chicken or tofu for a different protein source.

Why is this recipe good for PCOS?

This eggplant and chickpea stew is rich in fiber and plant-based protein, which help regulate blood sugar levels and promote satiety. The variety of spices not only adds flavor but also provides anti-inflammatory benefits. This dish is nutrient-dense, hearty, and perfect for a comforting meal for women managing PCOS.

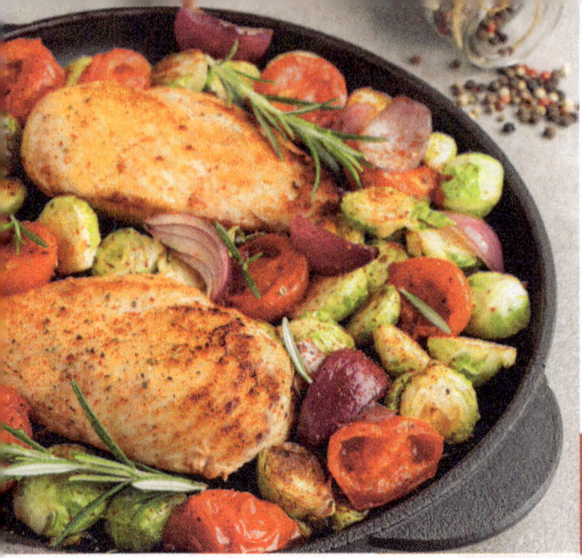

Lemon Herb Grilled Chicken with Roasted Brussels Sprouts

SERVING SIZE
Serves 2

INGREDIENTS

For the Chicken

- 2 boneless, skinless chicken breasts (about 6 ounces each)
- 2 tablespoons olive oil
- Juice of 1 lemon
- 2 cloves garlic, minced
- 1 teaspoon dried oregano
- 1 teaspoon dried thyme
- Salt and pepper to taste

For the Roasted Brussels Sprouts

- 2 cups Brussels sprouts, halved
- 1 tablespoon olive oil
- Salt and pepper to taste
- *Optional* 1 teaspoon balsamic vinegar for drizzling

DIRECTIONS

1. **Marinate Chicken:** In a bowl, whisk together olive oil, lemon juice, minced garlic, oregano, thyme, salt, and pepper. Add the chicken breasts and coat well. Marinate for at least 30 minutes (or up to 2 hours in the refrigerator).
2. **Preheat Oven:** Preheat your oven to 400°F (200°C).
3. **Prepare Brussels Sprouts:** On a baking sheet, toss the halved Brussels sprouts with olive oil, salt, and pepper. Spread them out in a single layer.
4. **Roast Brussels Sprouts:** Place the baking sheet in the preheated oven and roast for about 20-25 minutes, or until the Brussels sprouts are tender and golden brown, stirring halfway through.
5. **Grill Chicken:** While the Brussels sprouts are roasting, preheat a grill or grill pan over medium-high heat. Remove the chicken from the marinade and grill for about 6-7 minutes on each side, or until fully cooked and no longer pink in the center.
6. **Serve:** Once the chicken is cooked and the Brussels sprouts are roasted, plate the chicken alongside the Brussels sprouts. Drizzle with balsamic vinegar if desired.

Nutrition Information (Per Serving)

Calories	400
Protein	35g
Carbohydrates	15g
Dietary Fiber	6g
Sugars	3g
Fat	25g
Saturated Fat	4g

"Your journey is your power."

QUICK NOTES

TIPS FOR CUSTOMIZATION

- **Add More Veggies:** Include other vegetables like carrots, sweet potatoes, or bell peppers to roast alongside the Brussels sprouts.
- **Spice it Up:** Add red pepper flakes or a dash of hot sauce to the marinade for extra heat.
- **Herb Variations:** Experiment with different herbs like rosemary or basil for varied flavors.

Why is this recipe good for PCOS?

This dish is high in protein from the grilled chicken, which helps regulate blood sugar levels and promotes satiety. The Brussels sprouts provide fiber and essential nutrients while being low in carbohydrates. The healthy fats from olive oil support hormone balance, making this meal nutritious and satisfying for women managing PCOS.

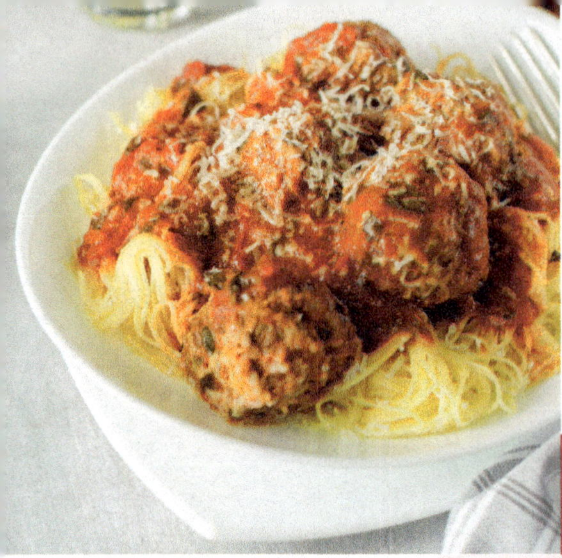

Spaghetti Squash with Meatballs and Marinara Sauce

SERVING SIZE
Serves 4

INGREDIENTS

For the Spaghetti Squash

- 1 medium spaghetti squash
- 1 tablespoon olive oil
- Salt and pepper to taste

For the Meatballs

- 1 pound ground turkey or lean ground beef
- 1/4 cup almond flour (or gluten-free breadcrumbs)
- 1/4 cup fresh parsley, chopped
- 1 egg, beaten
- 2 cloves garlic, minced
- 1 teaspoon Italian seasoning
- Salt and pepper to taste

For the Marinara Sauce

- 1 can (14 oz) marinara sauce (sugar-free if possible)
- 1 teaspoon dried oregano
- 1 teaspoon garlic powder
- Salt and pepper to taste

DIRECTIONS

1. **Preheat Oven:** Preheat your oven to 400°F (200°C).
2. **Prepare Spaghetti Squash:** Cut the spaghetti squash in half lengthwise and scoop out the seeds. Drizzle the inside with olive oil and season with salt and pepper. Place the squash cut-side down on a baking sheet and roast in the preheated oven for about 30-40 minutes, or until tender.
3. **Make Meatballs:** In a large bowl, combine the ground turkey (or beef), almond flour, parsley, beaten egg, minced garlic, Italian seasoning, salt, and pepper. Mix until well combined. Form the mixture into meatballs, about 1-2 inches in diameter.
4. **Cook Meatballs:** In a skillet over medium heat, add a little olive oil and cook the meatballs for about 5-7 minutes, turning occasionally, until browned on all sides. Remove from heat.
5. **Prepare Marinara Sauce:** In a saucepan, heat the marinara sauce over medium heat. Stir in the dried oregano, garlic powder, salt, and pepper. Let it simmer for a few minutes.
6. **Combine:** Once the spaghetti squash is cooked, remove it from the oven and let it cool slightly. Use a fork to scrape the flesh into spaghetti-like strands. Serve the spaghetti squash topped with meatballs and marinara sauce.
7. **Serve:** Garnish with additional parsley if desired and serve warm.

Nutrition Information (Per Serving)

Calories	350
Protein	30g
Carbohydrates	20g
Dietary Fiber	6g
Sugars	4g
Fat	18g
Saturated Fat	4g

"Be bold, be brave."

QUICK NOTES

TIPS FOR CUSTOMIZATION

- **Add Veggies:** Include sautéed spinach, mushrooms, or bell peppers in the marinara sauce for added nutrition.
- **Spice it Up:** Add red pepper flakes to the marinara sauce for extra heat.
- **Cheese Variations:** Top with nutritional yeast or dairy-free cheese for a cheesy flavor without dairy.

Why is this recipe good for PCOS?

This dish is low in carbohydrates and high in protein, making it an excellent choice for managing blood sugar levels. Spaghetti squash is a low-calorie, nutrient-dense alternative to traditional pasta, while the meatballs provide lean protein. The healthy fats from olive oil support hormone balance, making this meal nutritious and satisfying for women managing PCOS.

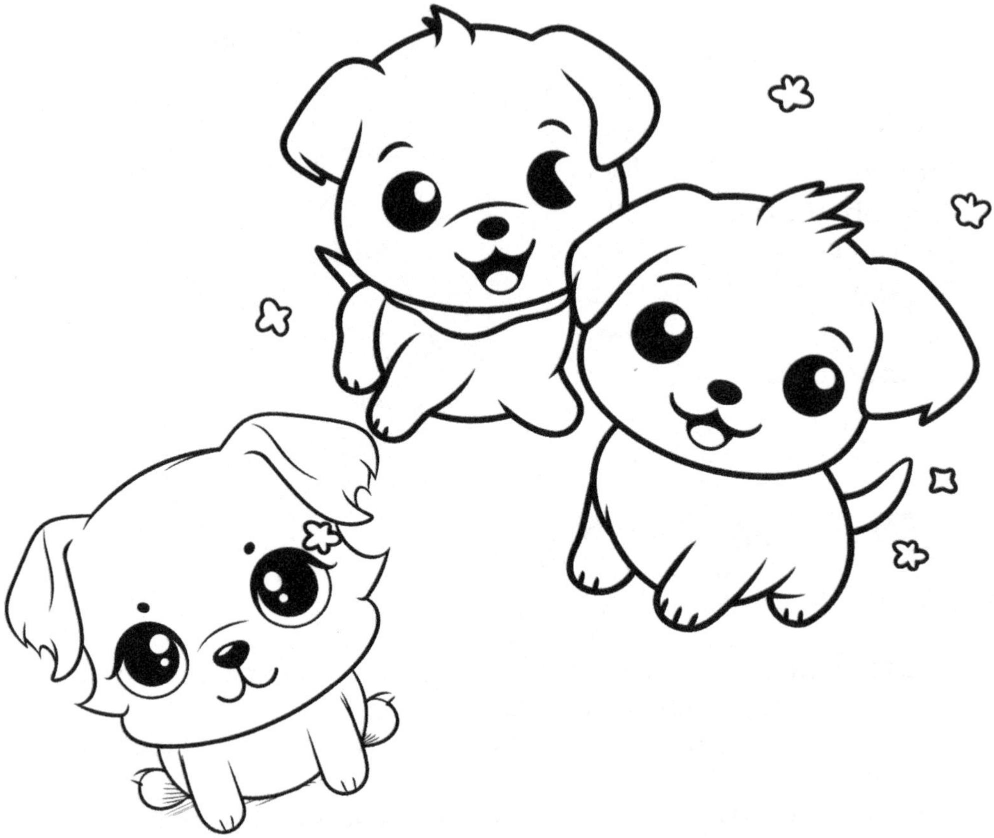

while I am able to manage my PCOS symptoms at this point in my life, I am still in a constant battle as most of us are. Fertility is still something I wish I have a secret formula for... we are still dearly praying and desiring for a child.

But we do have our 3 adorable furbabies at home with us - Frappu, Sasha, and their son Loki (we had sasha spayed when we decided to keep loki). We bring them with us even to our weekly trips to my parents' house for the weekends. They're a mix of mischief and unconditional love that I am so grateful to God for.

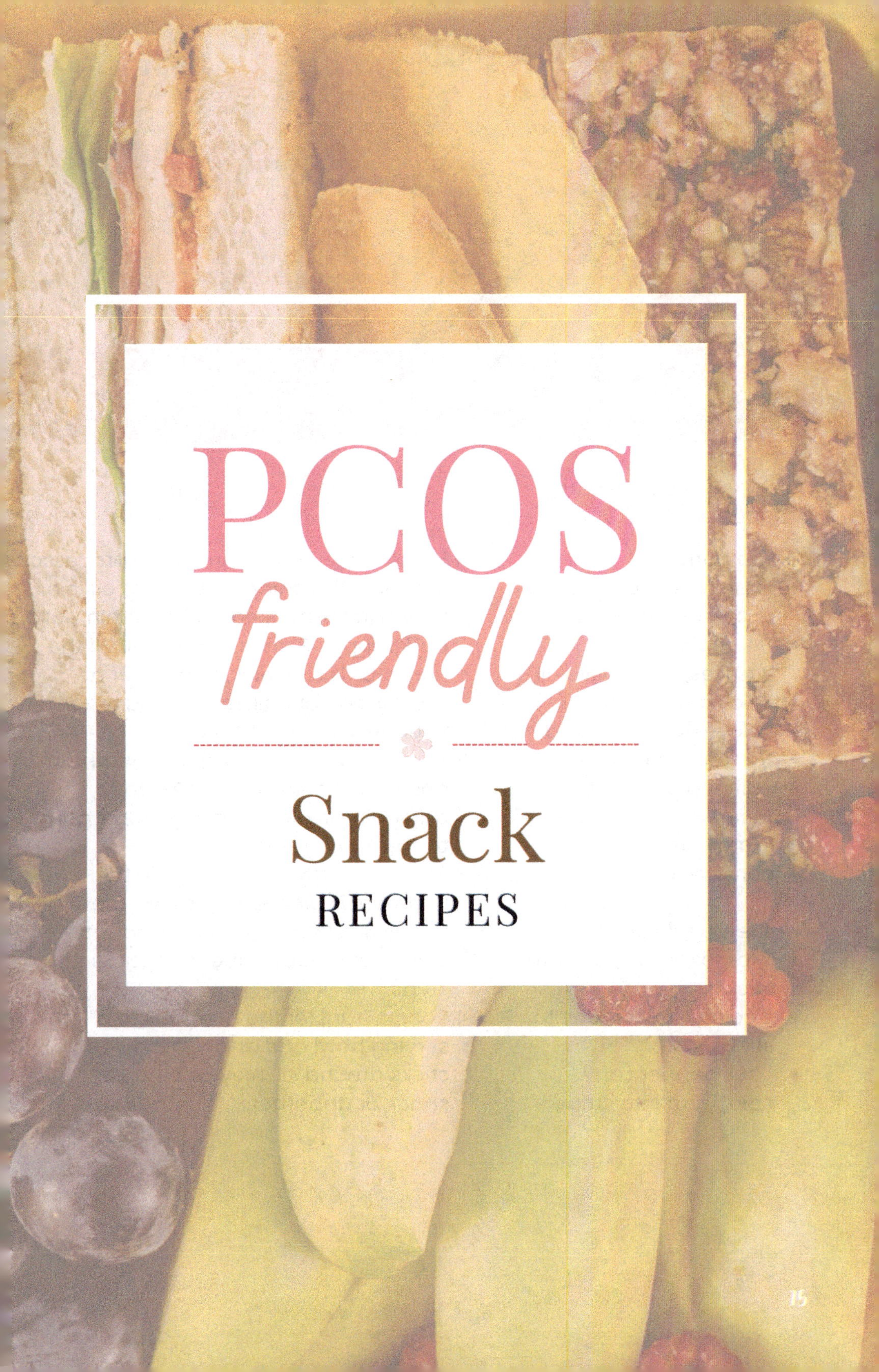

PCOS *friendly*

Snack

RECIPES

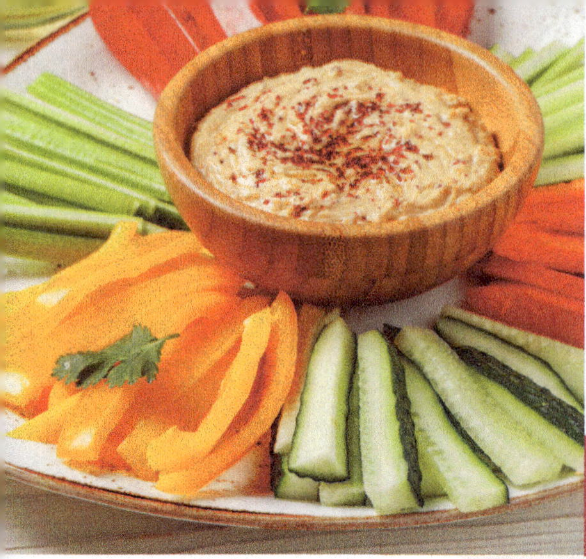

Hummus with Veggie Sticks (carrots, celery, bell peppers)

SERVING SIZE
Serves 4

INGREDIENTS

For the Hummus

- 1 can (15 oz) chickpeas, rinsed and drained
- 1/4 cup tahini
  2 tablespoons olive oil
- Juice of 1 lemon
- 1 clove garlic, minced
- 1/2 teaspoon cumin
- Salt and pepper to taste
- Water (as needed for consistency)

For the Veggie Sticks

- 2 large carrots, cut into sticks
- 2 celery stalks, cut into sticks
- 1 bell pepper (any color), cut into strips

DIRECTIONS

1. **Make the Hummus:** In a food processor, combine the chickpeas, tahini, olive oil, lemon juice, minced garlic, cumin, salt, and pepper. Blend until smooth. If the hummus is too thick, add water a tablespoon at a time until you reach your desired consistency.
2. **Taste and Adjust:** Taste the hummus and adjust seasoning as needed, adding more salt, lemon juice, or garlic to suit your preference.
3. **Prepare Veggie Sticks:** While the hummus is blending, prepare the veggie sticks by cutting the carrots, celery, and bell pepper into sticks or strips.
4. **Serve:** Transfer the hummus to a serving bowl and arrange the veggie sticks around it. Enjoy as a healthy snack or appetizer.

Nutrition Information (Per Serving)

Calories	150
Protein	5g
Carbohydrates	20g
Dietary Fiber	6g
Sugars	3g
Fat	7g
Saturated Fat	1g

"You are the author of your life."

QUICK NOTES

TIPS FOR CUSTOMIZATION

- **Add Flavor:** Mix in roasted red peppers, sun-dried tomatoes, or herbs like parsley or cilantro for different flavor profiles.
- **Spice it Up:** Add a pinch of cayenne pepper or smoked paprika for a spicy kick.
- **Nut Variations:** Substitute tahini with almond butter or sunflower seed butter for a different taste.

Why is this recipe good for PCOS?

Hummus is rich in plant-based protein and fiber, which help regulate blood sugar levels and promote satiety. The healthy fats from olive oil support hormone balance, while the variety of fresh vegetables provides essential vitamins and minerals. This snack is nutritious, satisfying, and perfect for women managing PCOS.

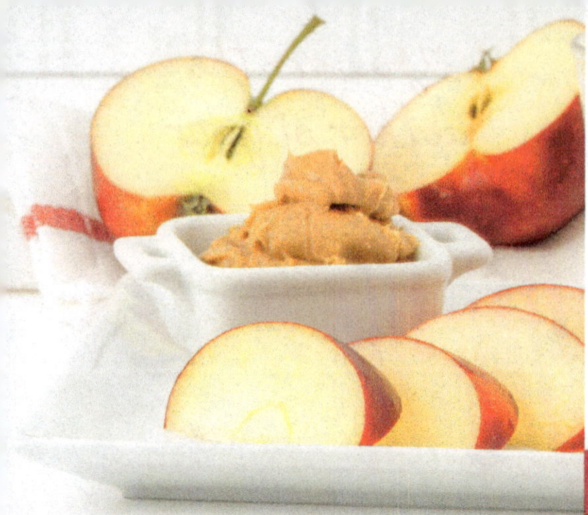

Apple Slices with Almond Butter

SERVING SIZE
Serves 1

INGREDIENTS

- 1 large apple (any variety, such as Fuji, Honeycrisp, or Granny Smith)
- 2 tablespoons almond butter (unsweetened)
- *Optional* Cinnamon for sprinkling
- *Optional* Chopped nuts or seeds for topping

DIRECTIONS

1. **Prepare Apple:** Wash the apple thoroughly. Core the apple and slice it into thin wedges or rounds.
2. **Serve with Almond Butter:** Arrange the apple slices on a plate and serve with almond butter on the side for dipping.
3. **Optional Toppings:** If desired, sprinkle cinnamon over the apple slices or top with chopped nuts or seeds for added crunch and flavor.

Nutrition Information (Per Serving)

Calories	200
Protein	4g
Carbohydrates	25g
Dietary Fiber	5g
Sugars	18g
Fat	10g
Saturated Fat	1g

"Strength is beauty."

QUICK NOTES

TIPS FOR CUSTOMIZATION

- **Add Flavor:** Mix in a dash of vanilla extract into the almond butter for extra flavor.
- **Fruit Variations:** Substitute apples with other fruits like pears or bananas for variety.
- **Nut Variations:** Use other nut butters like peanut butter or cashew butter if preferred.

Why is this recipe good for PCOS?

This snack is a great combination of fiber from the apple and healthy fats from almond butter, which helps regulate blood sugar levels and promotes satiety. The natural sugars in the apple provide a quick energy boost without causing spikes in blood sugar. This simple and nutritious snack is perfect for women managing PCOS.

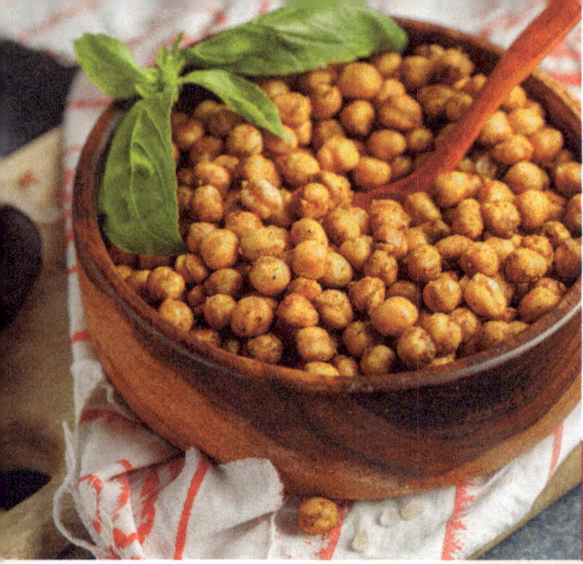

Roasted Chickpeas with Spices

SERVING SIZE
Serves 4 (1/2 cup per serving)

INGREDIENTS

- 1 can (15 oz) chickpeas, rinsed and drained
- 1 tablespoon olive oil
- 1 teaspoon smoked paprika
- 1 teaspoon cumin
- 1/2 teaspoon garlic powder
- 1/2 teaspoon onion powder
- 1/2 teaspoon salt
- 1/4 teaspoon black pepper
- *Optional*
  1/4 teaspoon cayenne pepper for heat

DIRECTIONS

1. **Preheat Oven:** Preheat your oven to 400°F (200°C).
2. **Prepare Chickpeas:** After rinsing and draining the chickpeas, pat them dry with a paper towel to remove excess moisture. This helps them become crispy when roasted.
3. **Season Chickpeas:** In a bowl, toss the chickpeas with olive oil, smoked paprika, cumin, garlic powder, onion powder, salt, black pepper, and cayenne pepper (if using) until evenly coated.
4. **Roast Chickpeas:** Spread the seasoned chickpeas in a single layer on a baking sheet. Roast in the preheated oven for about 25-30 minutes, stirring halfway through, until they are golden brown and crispy.
5. **Cool and Serve:** Remove from the oven and let them cool slightly. They will continue to crisp up as they cool. Enjoy as a healthy snack or topping for salads and bowls.

Nutrition Information (Per Serving)

Calories	150
Protein	7g
Carbohydrates	22g
Dietary Fiber	6g
Sugars	2g
Fat	5g
Saturated Fat	1g

"You are not alone."

QUICK NOTES

TIPS FOR CUSTOMIZATION

- **Add Flavor:** Experiment with different spices such as curry powder, chili powder, or Italian seasoning for varied flavors.
- **Sweet Option:** For a sweet version, toss with cinnamon and a touch of maple syrup before roasting.
- **Storage:** Store any leftovers in an airtight container at room temperature for up to 3 days. They may lose some crispiness over time.

Why is this recipe good for PCOS?

Roasted chickpeas are a great source of plant-based protein and fiber, which help regulate blood sugar levels and promote satiety. The spices add flavor without extra calories, making this a nutritious and satisfying snack for women managing PCOS. This recipe is easy to prepare and can be customized to suit your taste preferences.

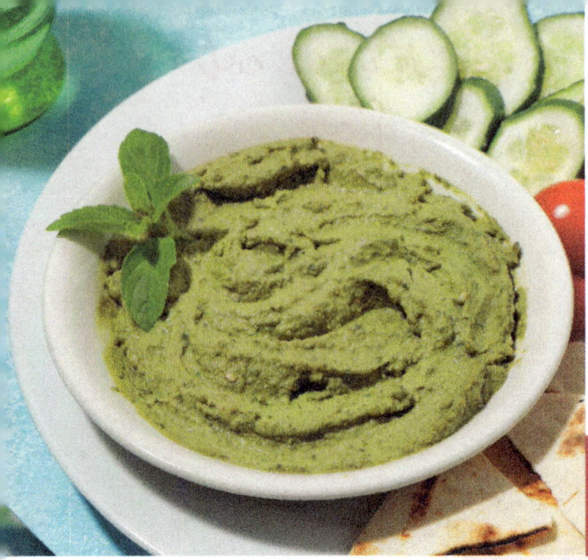

Guacamole with Cucumber Slices

SERVING SIZE
Serves 2-4 (depending on portion si

INGREDIENTS

For the Guacamole

- 2 ripe avocados
- Juice of 1 lime
- 1 small tomato, diced
- 1/4 small red onion, finely diced
- 1 clove garlic, minced
- 1/4 teaspoon cumin (optional)
- Salt and pepper to taste
- Optional
  Fresh cilantro, chopped, for garnish

For Serving

- 1 large cucumber, sliced into rounds or sticks

DIRECTIONS

1. **Prepare Guacamole:** In a medium bowl, scoop the flesh of the avocados and mash it with a fork until smooth or to your desired consistency.
2. **Add Ingredients:** Stir in the lime juice, diced tomato, red onion, minced garlic, cumin (if using), salt, and pepper. Mix until well combined. Taste and adjust seasoning as needed.
3. **Garnish:** If desired, garnish with chopped fresh cilantro.
4. **Serve:** Arrange cucumber slices on a plate and serve with the guacamole for dipping.

Nutrition Information (Per Serving)

Calories	150
Protein	2g
Carbohydrates	10g
Dietary Fiber	6g
Sugars	1g
Fat	12g
Saturated Fat	2g

"Dare to be different."

QUICK NOTES

TIPS FOR CUSTOMIZATION

- **Add Heat:** Include diced jalapeños or a dash of hot sauce for a spicy kick.
- **Flavor Variations:** Mix in diced bell peppers or corn for added texture and flavor.
- **Nut Variations:** Serve with other veggie sticks like carrots or bell peppers for variety.

Why is this recipe good for PCOS?

Guacamole is rich in healthy fats from avocados, which help regulate blood sugar levels and promote satiety. The fiber from cucumbers and avocados aids in digestion and helps maintain a healthy weight. This snack is nutritious, satisfying, and perfect for women managing PCOS, providing a delicious way to enjoy healthy fats and fresh vegetables.

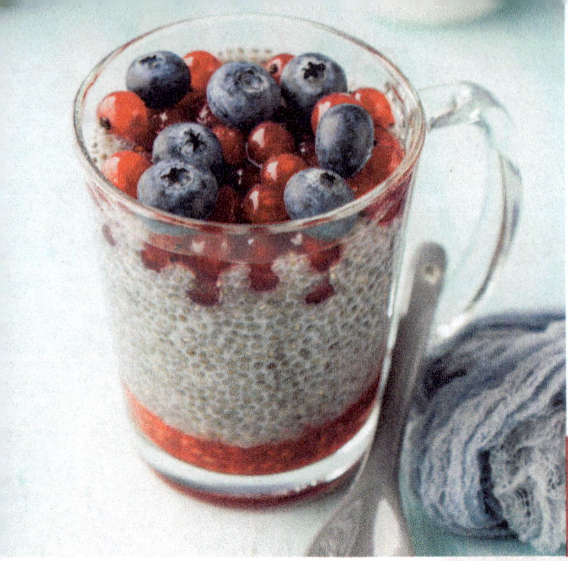

Chia Seed Pudding with Berries

SERVING SIZE
Serves 1

INGREDIENTS

- 1/4 cup chia seeds
- 1 cup unsweetened almond milk (or any dairy-free milk)
- 1 tablespoon maple syrup or a low-carb sweetener (like stevia or monk fruit) to taste
- 1/2 teaspoon vanilla extract (optional)
- 1/2 cup mixed berries (fresh or frozen, such as strawberries, blueberries, or raspberries)
- *Optional*
  Nuts or seeds for topping

DIRECTIONS

1. **Mix Ingredients:** In a bowl or jar, combine chia seeds, almond milk, maple syrup (or sweetener), and vanilla extract (if using). Stir well to ensure the chia seeds are evenly distributed.
2. **Refrigerate:** Cover the bowl or jar and refrigerate for at least 4 hours or overnight. The chia seeds will absorb the liquid and thicken to a pudding-like consistency.
3. **Stir and Serve:** After chilling, stir the pudding to break up any clumps. Top with mixed berries and nuts or seeds if desired before serving.

Nutrition Information (Per Serving)

Calories	250
Protein	6g
Carbohydrates	20g
Dietary Fiber	15g
Sugars	5g
Fat	16g
Saturated Fat	1g

"Your happiness matters."

QUICK NOTES

TIPS FOR CUSTOMIZATION

- **Flavor Variations:** Add a pinch of cinnamon or cocoa powder for different flavor profiles.
- **Fruit Options:** Use any seasonal fruits or your favorite berries for topping.
- **Nut Milk Alternatives:** Substitute almond milk with coconut milk or any other dairy-free milk of your choice.

Why is this recipe good for PCOS?

Chia seeds are an excellent source of omega-3 fatty acids, fiber, and protein, which help regulate blood sugar levels and promote satiety. The high fiber content aids in digestion and can help manage weight, which is beneficial for women with PCOS. This pudding is low in refined sugars and high in nutrients, making it a delicious and healthy breakfast or snack option.

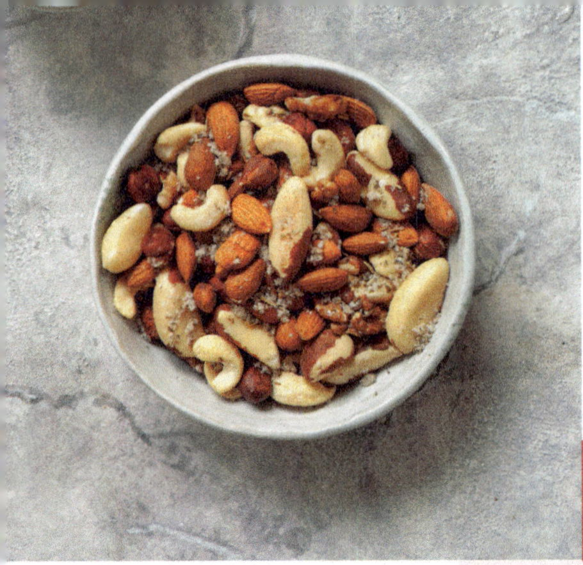

Nut and Seed Trail Mix (unsweetened and without added sugars)

SERVING SIZE
Serves 4 (1/4 cup per serving)

INGREDIENTS

- 1/2 cup raw almonds
- 1/2 cup raw walnuts
- 1/2 cup raw pumpkin seeds (pepitas)
- 1/2 cup raw sunflower seeds
- 1/4 cup unsweetened coconut flakes (optional)
- 1/4 teaspoon sea salt (optional)
- *Optional*
  1/4 cup dried unsweetened fruit (like cranberries or raisins) for sweetness

DIRECTIONS

1. **Combine Ingredients:** In a large bowl, combine the almonds, walnuts, pumpkin seeds, sunflower seeds, and coconut flakes (if using).
2. **Add Salt:** If desired, sprinkle with sea salt and mix well to combine.
3. **Store:** Transfer the trail mix to an airtight container or resealable bag for storage. It can be kept at room temperature for up to 2 weeks.

Nutrition Information (Per Serving)

Calories	200
Protein	6g
Carbohydrates	8g
Dietary Fiber	4g
Sugars	1g
Fat	18g
Saturated Fat	2g

"You are resilient."

QUICK NOTES

TIPS FOR CUSTOMIZATION

- **Add Flavor:** Mix in spices like cinnamon or a pinch of cayenne pepper for added flavor.
- **Nut Variations:** Substitute or add other nuts like pecans, cashews, or hazelnuts for variety.
- **Seed Variations:** Include chia seeds or flaxseeds for extra nutrition.

Why is this recipe good for PCOS?

This nut and seed trail mix is rich in healthy fats, protein, and fiber, which help regulate blood sugar levels and promote satiety. The combination of nuts and seeds provides essential vitamins and minerals, making it a nutritious and satisfying snack for women managing PCOS. This trail mix is easy to prepare and perfect for on-the-go snacking.

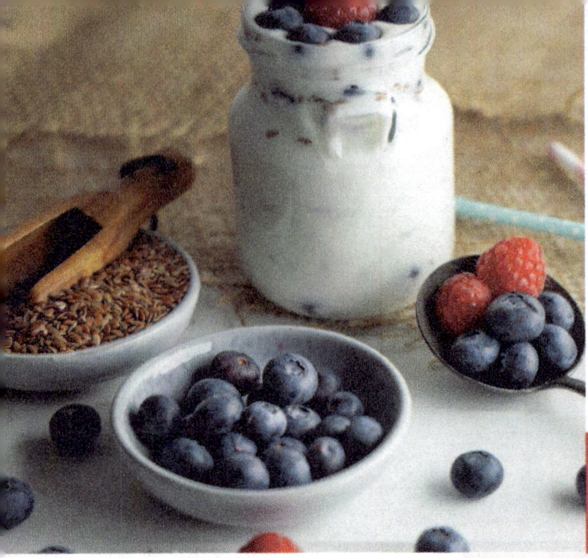

Coconut Yogurt with Flaxseeds and Berries

SERVING SIZE
Serves 1

INGREDIENTS

- 1 cup unsweetened coconut yogurt (dairy-free)
- 2 tablespoons ground flaxseeds
- 1/2 cup mixed berries (fresh or frozen, such as strawberries, blueberries, or raspberries)
- *Optional*
  1 tablespoon unsweetened shredded coconut for topping
- *Optional*
  1 tablespoon almond butter or nut butter of choice for added flavor

DIRECTIONS

1. **Prepare Yogurt Base:** In a bowl, add the coconut yogurt and mix in the ground flaxseeds until well combined.
2. **Add Berries:** Gently fold in the mixed berries, reserving a few for topping if desired.
3. **Serve:** Transfer the yogurt mixture to a serving bowl. Top with the reserved berries, shredded coconut, and almond butter (if using).
4. **Enjoy:** Serve immediately as a nutritious breakfast or snack.

Nutrition Information (Per Serving)

Calories	300
Protein	6g
Carbohydrates	30g
Dietary Fiber	10g
Sugars	5g
Fat	18g
Saturated Fat	15g

"Lift each other up."

QUICK NOTES

TIPS FOR CUSTOMIZATION

- **Add Flavor:** Mix in a dash of vanilla extract or cinnamon for extra flavor.
- **Nut Variations:** Substitute flaxseeds with chia seeds or hemp seeds for variety.
- **Sweetness:** If desired, add a low-carb sweetener like stevia or monk fruit to taste.

Why is this recipe good for PCOS?

This dish is rich in healthy fats from coconut yogurt and flaxseeds, which help regulate blood sugar levels and promote satiety. The fiber from flaxseeds and berries aids in digestion and can help manage weight, which is beneficial for women with PCOS. This recipe is nutrient-dense, delicious, and perfect for a healthy breakfast or snack option.

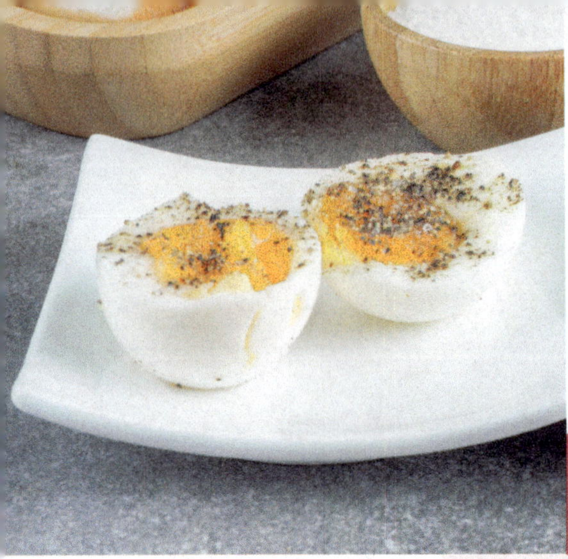

Hard-Boiled Eggs with Salt and Pepper

SERVING SIZE
Serves 2 (2 eggs per serving)

INGREDIENTS

- 4 large eggs
- Salt to taste
- Pepper to taste
- *Optional*
  Fresh herbs (like chives or parsley) for garnish

DIRECTIONS

1. **Boil the Eggs:** Place the eggs in a single layer in a saucepan and cover them with cold water, about an inch above the eggs. Bring the water to a boil over medium-high heat.
2. **Cook the Eggs:** Once the water reaches a rolling boil, cover the saucepan with a lid and remove it from heat. Let the eggs sit in the hot water for about 9-12 minutes, depending on how well-done you prefer the yolks (9 minutes for slightly soft yolks, 12 minutes for fully hard-boiled).
3. **Cool the Eggs:** After the cooking time is up, carefully transfer the eggs to a bowl of ice water or run them under cold water for a few minutes to stop the cooking process.
4. **Peel the Eggs:** Once cooled, gently tap the eggs on a hard surface to crack the shell, then peel under running water for easier removal.
5. **Season and Serve:** Slice the eggs in half or leave them whole. Sprinkle with salt and pepper to taste. Garnish with fresh herbs if desired.

Nutrition Information (Per Serving)

Calories	140
Protein	12g
Carbohydrates	1g
Dietary Fiber	0g
Sugars	0g
Fat	10g
Saturated Fat	3g

"You are deserving of greatness."

QUICK NOTES

TIPS FOR CUSTOMIZATION

- **Add Flavor:** Mix in spices like paprika, cayenne pepper, or everything bagel seasoning for extra flavor.
- **Dipping Sauce:** Serve with a side of hummus or guacamole for dipping.
- **Salad Addition:** Chop the hard-boiled eggs and add them to salads for added protein.

Why is this recipe good for PCOS?

Hard-boiled eggs are an excellent source of high-quality protein and healthy fats, which help regulate blood sugar levels and promote satiety. They are low in carbohydrates, making them a great snack option for women managing PCOS. This simple recipe is nutritious, easy to prepare, and perfect for on-the-go snacking.

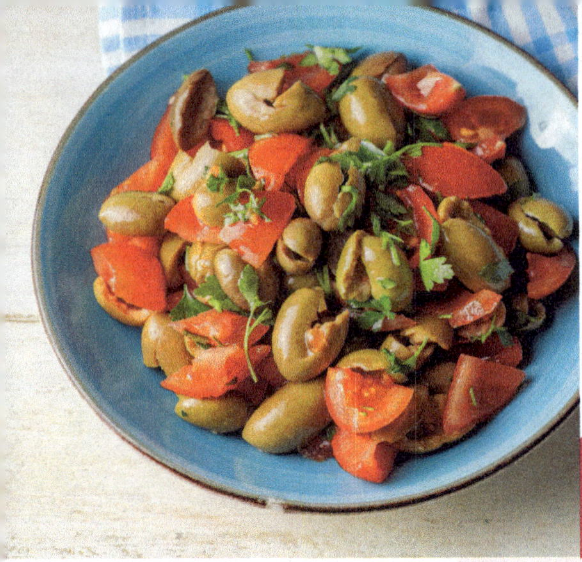

Olives and Cherry Tomatoes

SERVING SIZE
Serves 2

INGREDIENTS

- 1 cup mixed olives (green and black, pitted)
- 1 cup cherry tomatoes, halved
- 1 tablespoon olive oil
- 1 teaspoon dried oregano
  Salt and pepper to taste
- *Optional*
  Fresh basil or parsley for garnish
- *Optional*
  Balsamic vinegar for drizzling

DIRECTIONS

1. **Prepare Ingredients:** In a medium bowl, combine the mixed olives and halved cherry tomatoes.
2. **Season:** Drizzle with olive oil and sprinkle with dried oregano, salt, and pepper. Toss gently to combine and coat the olives and tomatoes evenly.
3. **Serve:** Transfer to a serving dish. If desired, garnish with fresh basil or parsley and drizzle with balsamic vinegar for added flavor.
4. **Enjoy:** Serve immediately as a healthy snack or appetizer.

Nutrition Information (Per Serving)

Calories	150
Protein	2g
Carbohydrates	8g
Dietary Fiber	2g
Sugars	2g
Fat	14g
Saturated Fat	2g

"Find joy in the journey."

QUICK NOTES

TIPS FOR CUSTOMIZATION

- **Add Flavor:** Mix in diced bell peppers or cucumbers for added crunch and nutrition.
- **Spice it Up:** Add red pepper flakes for a spicy kick.
- **Cheese Option:** Include crumbled feta or goat cheese for extra flavor (if dairy is acceptable).

Why is this recipe good for PCOS?

This simple dish is rich in healthy fats from olives, which help regulate blood sugar levels and promote satiety. The cherry tomatoes provide antioxidants and vitamins, making this a nutritious and satisfying snack for women managing PCOS. This recipe is quick to prepare and perfect for on-the-go snacking or as a light appetizer.

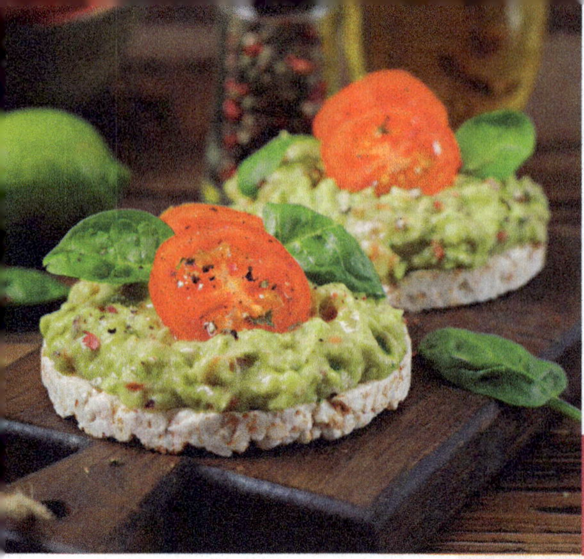

Rice Cakes with Avocado and Tomato

SERVING SIZE
Serves 1 (2 rice cakes)

INGREDIENTS

- 2 plain rice cakes (gluten-free if needed)
- 1 ripe avocado
- 1 medium tomato, sliced
- Salt and pepper to taste
- *Optional* Red pepper flakes for a spicy kick
- *Optional* Fresh herbs (like basil or cilantro) for garnish
- *Optional* Lemon juice for drizzling

DIRECTIONS

1. **Prepare Avocado:** In a bowl, mash the avocado with a fork until smooth. If desired, add a squeeze of lemon juice, salt, and pepper to taste.
2. **Assemble Rice Cakes:** Spread a generous layer of mashed avocado on each rice cake.
3. **Top with Tomato:** Place slices of tomato on top of the avocado spread.
4. **Season:** Sprinkle with additional salt, pepper, and red pepper flakes if desired. Garnish with fresh herbs for added flavor.
5. **Serve:** Enjoy immediately as a healthy snack or light meal.

Nutrition Information (Per Serving)

Calories	250
Protein	4g
Carbohydrates	30g
Dietary Fiber	8g
Sugars	2g
Fat	14g
Saturated Fat	2g

"Your dreams are within reach."

QUICK NOTES

TIPS FOR CUSTOMIZATION

- **Add Flavor:** Mix in spices like garlic powder or onion powder to the avocado for extra flavor.
- **Vegetable Variations:** Include sliced cucumbers or radishes for added crunch and nutrition.
- **Protein Boost:** Top with sliced hard-boiled eggs or smoked salmon for an extra protein boost.

Why is this recipe good for PCOS?

This dish is rich in healthy fats from avocado, which help regulate blood sugar levels and promote satiety. The fiber from rice cakes and vegetables aids in digestion and can help manage weight, which is beneficial for women with PCOS. This recipe is quick to prepare, nutritious, and perfect for a satisfying snack or light meal.

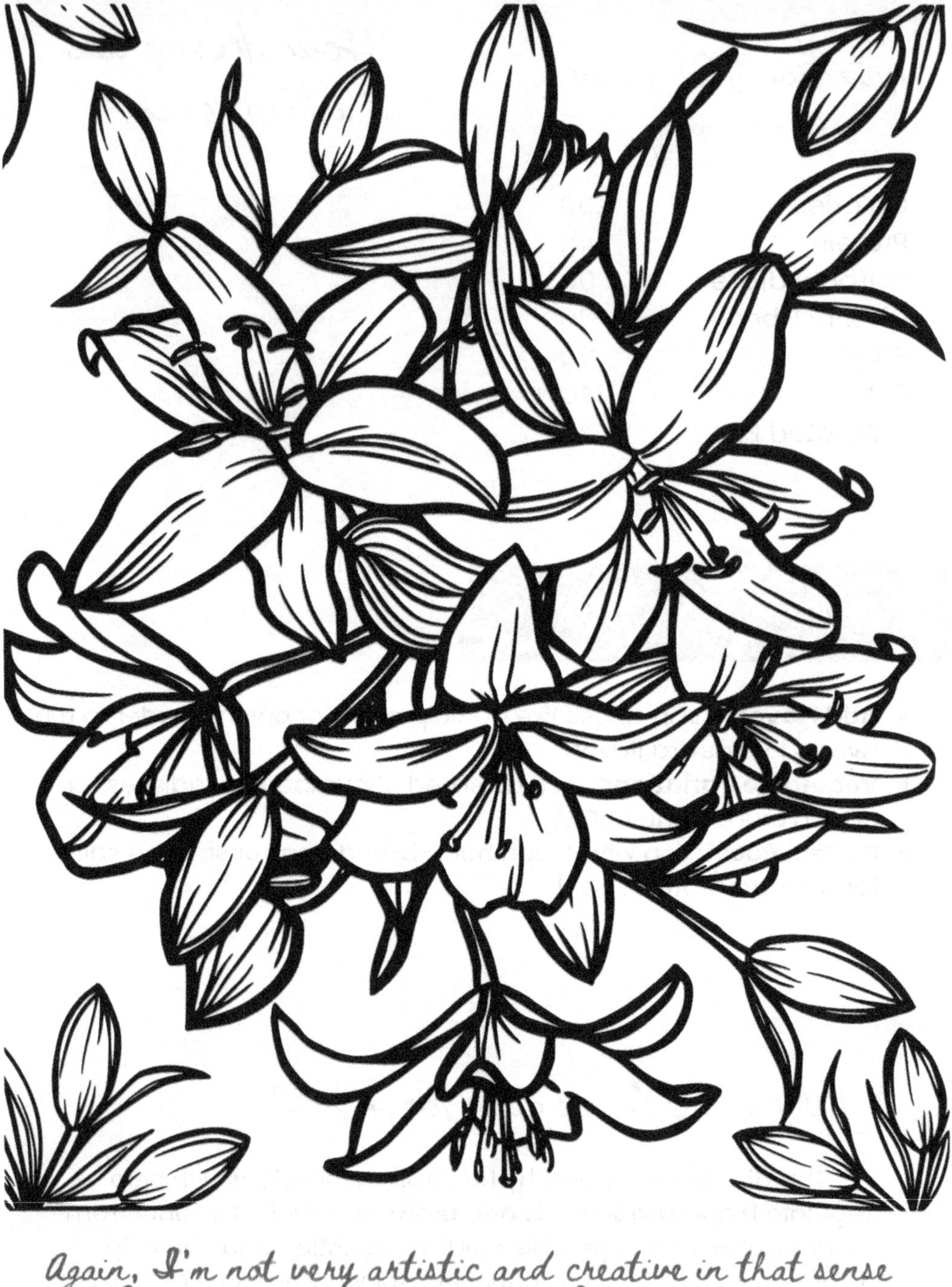

Again, I'm not very artistic and creative in that sense but I recently found a skill that I am getting good at – arranging the centerpiece flowers in church for the Sunday service.

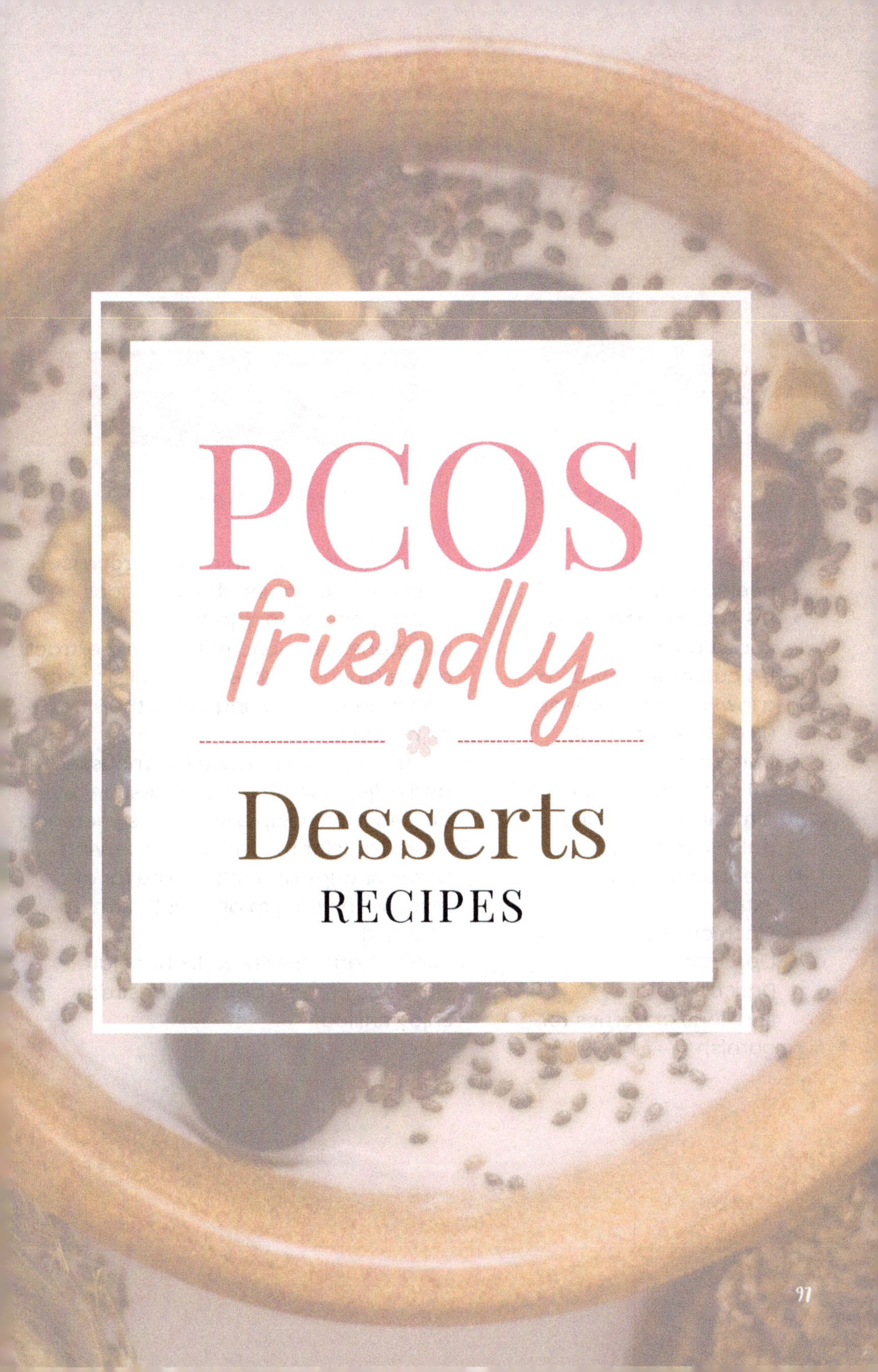

PCOS *friendly*

Desserts

RECIPES

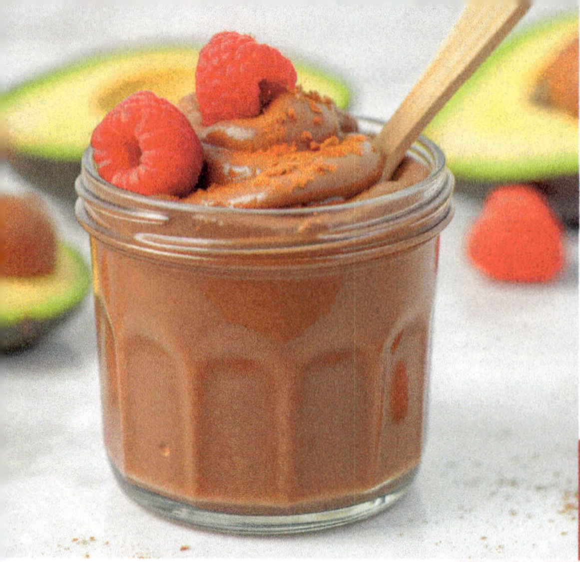

Dark Chocolate Avocado Mousse

SERVING SIZE
Serves 4

INGREDIENTS

- 2 ripe avocados, peeled and pitted
- 1/4 cup unsweetened cocoa powder
- 1/4 cup maple syrup or a low-carb sweetener (like stevia or monk fruit) to taste
- 1/4 cup unsweetened almond milk (or any dairy-free milk)
- 1 teaspoon vanilla extract
- Pinch of salt
- *Optional* Dark chocolate shavings or berries for garnish

DIRECTIONS

1. **Blend Ingredients:** In a food processor or blender, combine the avocados, cocoa powder, maple syrup (or sweetener), almond milk, vanilla extract, and a pinch of salt. Blend until smooth and creamy, scraping down the sides as needed.
2. **Taste and Adjust:** Taste the mousse and adjust sweetness if necessary by adding more maple syrup or sweetener.
3. **Chill:** Transfer the mousse to serving bowls or cups and refrigerate for at least 30 minutes to allow it to firm up and chill.
4. **Serve:** Garnish with dark chocolate shavings or fresh berries if desired. Enjoy chilled.

Nutrition Information (Per Serving)

Calories	180
Protein	3g
Carbohydrates	20g
Dietary Fiber	6g
Sugars	5g
Fat	10g
Saturated Fat	2g

"You are a beacon of hope."

QUICK NOTES

TIPS FOR CUSTOMIZATION

- **Add Flavor:** Mix in a pinch of cinnamon or a splash of espresso for added depth of flavor.
- **Nut Variations:** Top with chopped nuts or seeds for added crunch.
- **Sweetness Variations:** Adjust the sweetness based on your preference and the ripeness of the avocados.

Why is this recipe good for PCOS?

This dark chocolate avocado mousse is rich in healthy fats from avocados, which help regulate blood sugar levels and promote satiety. The cocoa powder provides antioxidants, while the natural sweetness from maple syrup or a low-carb sweetener keeps it low in refined sugars. This dessert is nutritious, satisfying, and a delicious way to enjoy a sweet treat while managing PCOS.

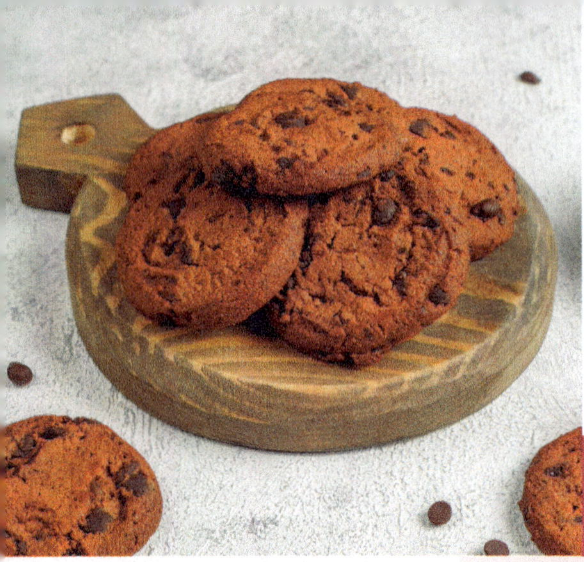

Coconut Flour Cookies with Dark Chocolate Chips

SERVING SIZE
Serves 8 (2 cookies per serving)

INGREDIENTS

- 1/2 cup coconut flour
- 1/4 cup coconut oil, melted (or unsalted butter)
- 1/4 cup maple syrup or a low-carb sweetener (like stevia or monk fruit)
- 2 large eggs
- 1/2 teaspoon vanilla extract
- 1/2 teaspoon baking soda
- 1/4 teaspoon salt
- 1/2 cup dark chocolate chips (dairy-free if needed)

DIRECTIONS

1. **Preheat Oven:** Preheat your oven to 350°F (175°C) and line a baking sheet with parchment paper.
2. **Mix Wet Ingredients:** In a large bowl, combine the melted coconut oil, maple syrup (or sweetener), eggs, and vanilla extract. Whisk until well combined.
3. **Add Dry Ingredients:** In another bowl, mix together the coconut flour, baking soda, and salt. Gradually add the dry ingredients to the wet ingredients, stirring until a dough forms. The dough will be thick.
4. **Fold in Chocolate Chips:** Gently fold in the dark chocolate chips until evenly distributed throughout the dough.
5. **Scoop Cookies:** Using a tablespoon or cookie scoop, drop rounded balls of dough onto the prepared baking sheet, spacing them about 2 inches apart. Flatten them slightly with the back of the scoop or your fingers.
6. **Bake:** Bake in the preheated oven for 10-12 minutes, or until the edges are lightly golden. The cookies will firm up as they cool.
7. **Cool and Serve:** Allow the cookies to cool on the baking sheet for a few minutes before transferring them to a wire rack to cool completely.

Nutrition Information (Per Serving)

Calories	180
Protein	3g
Carbohydrates	15g
Dietary Fiber	5g
Sugars	4g
Fat	12g
Saturated Fat	8g

"Embrace your inner goddess."

QUICK NOTES

TIPS FOR CUSTOMIZATION

- **Add Nuts:** Mix in chopped nuts like walnuts or pecans for added texture and flavor.
- **Flavor Variations:** Add a pinch of cinnamon or a splash of almond extract for different flavor profiles.
- **Sweetness Adjustments:** Adjust the sweetness based on your preference and the type of chocolate chips used.

Why is this recipe good for PCOS?

These coconut flour cookies are low in carbohydrates and high in fiber, making them a great option for managing blood sugar levels. The healthy fats from coconut oil and dark chocolate support hormone balance, while the use of coconut flour provides a gluten-free alternative. This dessert is nutritious, satisfying, and perfect for a sweet treat while managing PCOS.

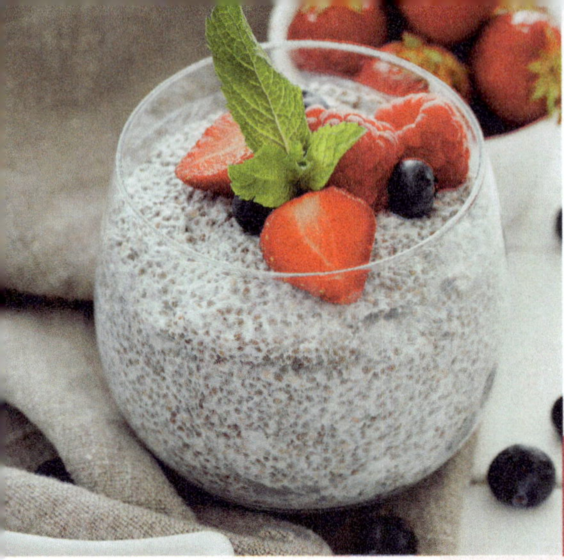

Chia Seed Pudding with Almond Milk and Berries

SERVING SIZE
Serves 1

INGREDIENTS

- 1/4 cup chia seeds
- 1 cup unsweetened almond milk (or any dairy-free milk)
- 1 tablespoon maple syrup or a low-carb sweetener (like stevia or monk fruit) to taste
- 1/2 teaspoon vanilla extract (optional)
- 1/2 cup mixed berries (fresh or frozen, such as strawberries, blueberries, or raspberries)
- *Optional*
  Nuts or seeds for topping

DIRECTIONS

1. **Mix Ingredients:** In a bowl or jar, combine chia seeds, almond milk, maple syrup (or sweetener), and vanilla extract (if using). Stir well to ensure the chia seeds are evenly distributed.
2. **Refrigerate:** Cover the bowl or jar and refrigerate for at least 4 hours or overnight. The chia seeds will absorb the liquid and thicken to a pudding-like consistency.
3. **Stir and Serve:** After chilling, stir the pudding to break up any clumps. Top with mixed berries and nuts or seeds if desired before serving.

Nutrition Information (Per Serving)

Calories	250
Protein	6g
Carbohydrates	20g
Dietary Fiber	15g
Sugars	5g
Fat	16g
Saturated Fat	1g

"You are capable of amazing things."

QUICK NOTES

TIPS FOR CUSTOMIZATION

- **Add Flavor:** Mix in a pinch of cinnamon or cocoa powder for different flavor profiles.
- **Fruit Options:** Use any seasonal fruits or your favorite berries for topping.
- **Nut Milk Alternatives:** Substitute almond milk with coconut milk or any other dairy-free milk of your choice.

Why is this recipe good for PCOS?

Chia seeds are an excellent source of omega-3 fatty acids, fiber, and protein, which help regulate blood sugar levels and promote satiety. The high fiber content aids in digestion and can help manage weight, which is beneficial for women with PCOS. This pudding is low in refined sugars and high in nutrients, making it a delicious and healthy breakfast or snack option.

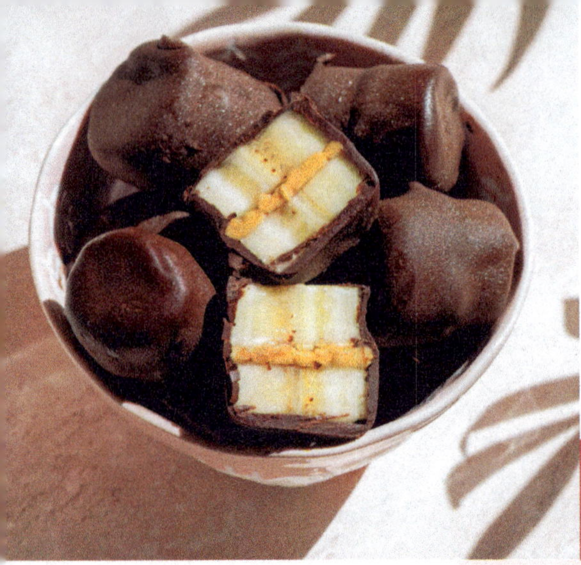

Frozen Banana Bites with Almond Butter

SERVING SIZE
Serves 4 (2-3 bites per serving)

INGREDIENTS

- 2 ripe bananas
- 1/2 cup almond butter (or any nut butter of your choice)
- 1/4 cup dark chocolate chips (dairy-free if needed)
- *Optional*
  Sea salt for sprinkling

DIRECTIONS

1. **Prepare Bananas:** Peel the bananas and slice them into 1/2-inch thick rounds.
2. **Spread Almond Butter:** On half of the banana slices, spread a small amount of almond butter. Top with the remaining banana slices to create little sandwiches.
3. **Melt Chocolate:** In a microwave-safe bowl, melt the dark chocolate chips in 30-second intervals, stirring in between until smooth.
4. **Dip Banana Bites:** Dip each banana sandwich into the melted chocolate, ensuring it is fully coated. Use a fork to lift it out and let any excess chocolate drip off.
5. **Freeze:** Place the chocolate-covered banana bites on a parchment-lined baking sheet. If desired, sprinkle with a pinch of sea salt before freezing. Freeze for at least 1-2 hours until solid.
6. **Serve:** Once frozen, transfer the banana bites to an airtight container and store in the freezer. Enjoy as a healthy snack or dessert!

Nutrition Information (Per Serving)

Calories	150
Protein	4g
Carbohydrates	20g
Dietary Fiber	3g
Sugars	8g
Fat	7g
Saturated Fat	1g

"Let your heart lead the way."

QUICK NOTES

TIPS FOR CUSTOMIZATION

- **Add Flavor:** Mix in a dash of cinnamon or vanilla extract into the almond butter for extra flavor.
- **Nut Variations:** Substitute almond butter with peanut butter, cashew butter, or sunflower seed butter.
- **Toppings:** Roll the banana bites in crushed nuts or seeds before freezing for added texture.

Why is this recipe good for PCOS?

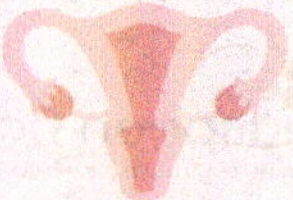

These frozen banana bites are a great source of healthy fats from almond butter, which help regulate blood sugar levels and promote satiety. The natural sugars from bananas provide a quick energy boost without causing spikes in blood sugar. This recipe is nutritious, easy to prepare, and perfect for a satisfying snack or dessert for women managing PCOS.

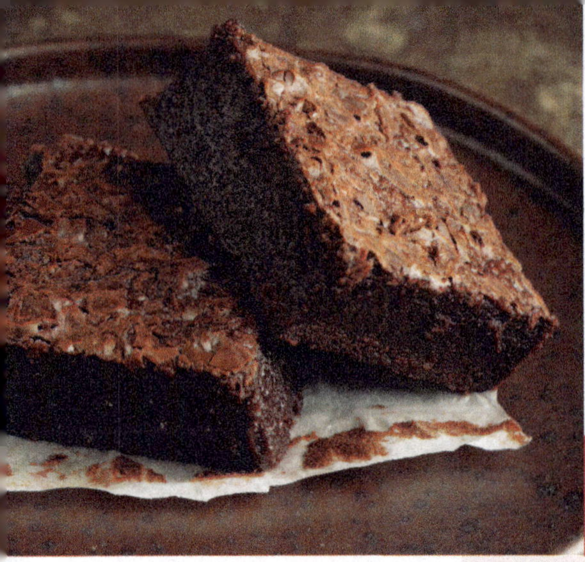

Almond Flour Brownies

SERVING SIZE
Serves 9 (1 brownie per serving)

INGREDIENTS

- 1 cup almond flour
- 1/2 cup unsweetened cocoa powder
- 1/2 cup maple syrup or a low-carb sweetener (like stevia or monk fruit)
- 1/4 cup coconut oil or unsalted butter, melted
- 2 large eggs
- 1 teaspoon vanilla extract
- 1/2 teaspoon baking soda
- 1/4 teaspoon salt
- *Optional*
  1/2 cup dark chocolate chips (dairy-free if needed) for added richness

DIRECTIONS

1. **Preheat Oven:** Preheat your oven to 350°F (175°C) and line an 8x8-inch baking pan with parchment paper or grease it lightly.
2. **Mix Wet Ingredients:** In a large mixing bowl, combine the melted coconut oil (or butter), maple syrup (or sweetener), eggs, and vanilla extract. Whisk until well combined.
3. **Add Dry Ingredients:** In another bowl, mix together the almond flour, cocoa powder, baking soda, and salt. Gradually add the dry ingredients to the wet ingredients, stirring until just combined. If using, fold in the dark chocolate chips.
4. **Pour into Pan:** Pour the brownie batter into the prepared baking pan and spread it evenly.
5. **Bake:** Bake in the preheated oven for about 20-25 minutes, or until a toothpick inserted into the center comes out mostly clean (a few moist crumbs are okay).
6. **Cool and Serve:** Allow the brownies to cool in the pan for about 10 minutes before transferring them to a wire rack to cool completely. Cut into squares and serve.

Nutrition Information (Per Serving)

Calories	180
Protein	5g
Carbohydrates	15g
Dietary Fiber	3g
Sugars	5g
Fat	12g
Saturated Fat	4g

"You are fierce and fabulous."

QUICK NOTES

TIPS FOR CUSTOMIZATION

- **Add Nuts:** Mix in chopped walnuts or pecans for added texture and flavor.
- **Flavor Variations:** Add a pinch of cinnamon or espresso powder for a richer chocolate flavor.
- **Frosting Option:** Top with a simple chocolate ganache made from melted dark chocolate and coconut cream for an indulgent treat.

Why is this recipe good for PCOS?

These almond flour brownies are low in carbohydrates and high in healthy fats, making them a great option for managing blood sugar levels. Almond flour provides protein and fiber, while cocoa powder offers antioxidants. This dessert is nutritious, satisfying, and perfect for a sweet treat while managing PCOS.

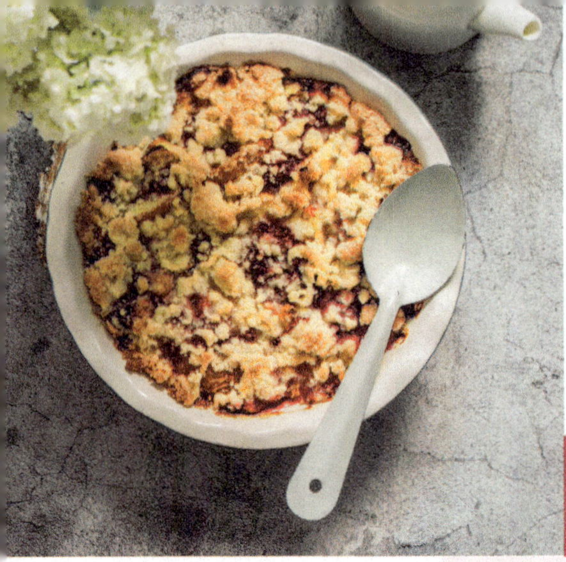

Berry Crumble with Oat Topping

SERVING SIZE
Serves 4

INGREDIENTS

For the Berry Filling

- 2 cups mixed berries (fresh or frozen, such as blueberries, raspberries, and strawberries)
- 2 tablespoons maple syrup or a low-carb sweetener (like stevia or mon) to taste
- 1 tablespoon cornstarch or arrowroot powder (for thickening)
- 1 teaspoon vanilla extract

For the Oat Topping

- 1 cup rolled oats (gluten-free if needed)
- 1/2 cup almond flour (or any flour of your choice)
- 1/4 cup coconut oil or unsalted butter, melted
- 1/4 cup maple syrup or a low-carb sweetener (like stevia or monk fruit)
- 1/2 teaspoon cinnamon
- Pinch of salt

DIRECTIONS

1. **Preheat Oven:** Preheat your oven to 350°F (175°C).
2. **Prepare Berry Filling:** In a mixing bowl, combine the mixed berries, maple syrup (or sweetener), cornstarch, and vanilla extract. Toss gently to coat the berries evenly. Transfer the mixture to a greased baking dish.
3. **Make Oat Topping:** In another bowl, combine the rolled oats, almond flour, melted coconut oil (or butter), maple syrup (or sweetener), cinnamon, and salt. Mix until crumbly and well combined.
4. **Assemble Crumble:** Evenly spread the oat topping over the berry filling in the baking dish.
5. **Bake:** Bake in the preheated oven for about 25-30 minutes, or until the topping is golden brown and the berries are bubbling.
6. **Serve:** Allow to cool slightly before serving. Enjoy warm, optionally topped with dairy-free yogurt or whipped coconut cream.

Nutrition Information (Per Serving)

Calories	250
Protein	4g
Carbohydrates	35g
Dietary Fiber	6g
Sugars	10g
Fat	12g
Saturated Fat	8g

"Your story inspires others."

QUICK NOTES

TIPS FOR CUSTOMIZATION

- **Add Nuts:** Mix in chopped nuts like walnuts or pecans for added crunch in the topping.
- **Fruit Variations:** Use any combination of fruits, such as peaches, apples, or cherries, for different flavors.
- **Spice it Up:** Add a pinch of nutmeg or ginger for extra warmth and flavor.

Why is this recipe good for PCOS?

This berry crumble is rich in fiber from the oats and berries, which helps regulate blood sugar levels and promotes satiety. The healthy fats from coconut oil or butter support hormone balance, while the natural sweetness from berries provides antioxidants and vitamins. This dessert is nutritious, satisfying, and perfect for a healthy treat while managing PCOS.

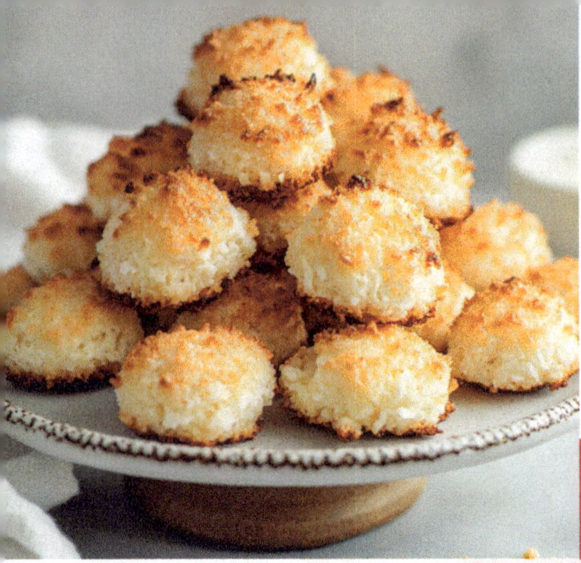

Coconut Macaroons with Sugar-Free Sweetener

SERVING SIZE
Serves 12 (1 macaroon per serving)

INGREDIENTS

- 2 1/2 cups unsweetened shredded coconut
- 1/4 cup sugar-free sweetener (like stevia, adjust to taste)
- 2 large egg whites
- 1 teaspoon vanilla extract
- 1/4 teaspoon salt
- *Optional*
  1/4 cup dark chocolate chips (dairy-free if needed) for drizzling

DIRECTIONS

1. **Preheat Oven:** Preheat your oven to 325°F (160°C) and line a baking sheet with parchment paper.
2. **Mix Ingredients:** In a large mixing bowl, combine the shredded coconut, sugar-free sweetener, egg whites, vanilla extract, and salt. Mix well until all ingredients are fully combined.
3. **Form Macaroons:** Using a tablespoon or cookie scoop, drop rounded mounds of the coconut mixture onto the prepared baking sheet, spacing them about 1 inch apart.
4. **Bake:** Bake in the preheated oven for about 15-20 minutes, or until the macaroons are golden brown on the edges. Keep an eye on them to prevent burning.
5. **Cool:** Remove from the oven and let the macaroons cool on the baking sheet for a few minutes before transferring them to a wire rack to cool completely.
6. **Optional Chocolate Drizzle:** If desired, melt the dark chocolate chips in a microwave-safe bowl in 30-second intervals, stirring until smooth. Drizzle over the cooled macaroons.

Nutrition Information (Per Serving)

Calories	120
Protein	2g
Carbohydrates	6g
Dietary Fiber	2g
Sugars	1g
Fat	10g
Saturated Fat	8g

"Keep shining, beautiful."

QUICK NOTES

TIPS FOR CUSTOMIZATION

- **Add Flavor:** Mix in a teaspoon of almond extract for a different flavor profile.
- **Nut Variations:** Add chopped nuts or seeds for added texture.
- **Storage:** Store in an airtight container at room temperature for up to a week or in the refrigerator for longer freshness.

Why is this recipe good for PCOS?

These coconut macaroons are low in carbohydrates and sugar, making them a great option for managing blood sugar levels. The healthy fats from coconut provide satiety, while the use of sugar-free sweetener helps keep the dessert low in calories. This recipe is simple, delicious, and perfect for a sweet treat while managing PCOS.

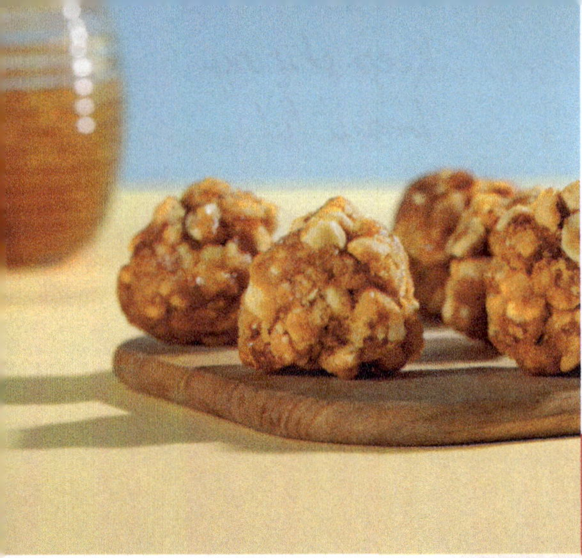

Peanut Butter Protein Balls

SERVING SIZE
Serves 8 (2 balls per serving)

INGREDIENTS

- 1 cup natural peanut butter (or any nut butter of your choice)
- 1/2 cup rolled oats (gluten-free if needed)
- 1/4 cup honey or a low-carb sweetener (like stevia or monk fruit) to taste
- 1/4 cup protein powder (vanilla or chocolate flavor)
- 1/4 cup ground flaxseeds (optional)
- 1/2 teaspoon vanilla extract
- *Optional*
  1/4 cup dark chocolate chips or chopped nuts for added texture

DIRECTIONS

1. **Mix Ingredients:** In a large mixing bowl, combine the peanut butter, rolled oats, honey (or sweetener), protein powder, ground flaxseeds (if using), and vanilla extract. Mix until well combined. If desired, fold in dark chocolate chips or chopped nuts.
2. **Form Balls:** Using your hands, scoop out small portions of the mixture and roll them into balls, about 1 inch in diameter. Place the balls on a parchment-lined baking sheet or plate.
3. **Chill:** Refrigerate the protein balls for at least 30 minutes to firm up.
4. **Serve:** Enjoy as a quick snack or post-workout treat. Store any leftovers in an airtight container in the refrigerator for up to a week.

Nutrition Information (Per Serving)

Calories	250
Protein	10g
Carbohydrates	20g
Dietary Fiber	4g
Sugars	5g
Fat	16g
Saturated Fat	3g

"You are a trailblazer."

QUICK NOTES

TIPS FOR CUSTOMIZATION

- **Add Flavor:** Mix in a pinch of cinnamon or cocoa powder for added flavor.
- **Nut Variations:** Substitute peanut butter with almond butter, cashew butter, or sunflower seed butter for variety.
- **Sweetness Adjustments:** Adjust the sweetness based on your preference and the type of protein powder used.

Why is this recipe good for PCOS?

These peanut butter protein balls are rich in healthy fats and protein, which help regulate blood sugar levels and promote satiety. The fiber from oats and flaxseeds aids in digestion and can help manage weight, which is beneficial for women with PCOS. This recipe is easy to prepare, nutritious, and perfect for a satisfying snack or post-workout treat.

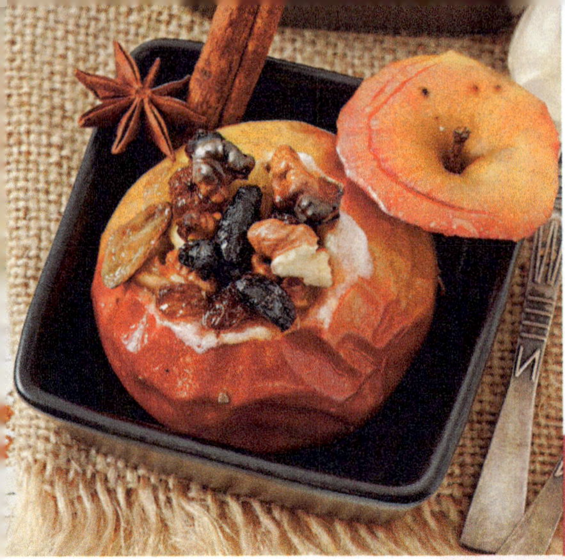

Baked Apples with Cinnamon and Walnuts

SERVING SIZE
Serves 4

INGREDIENTS

- 4 medium apples (such as Granny Smith or Honeycrisp)
- 1/2 cup walnuts, chopped
- 1/4 cup raisins or dried cranberries (optional)
- 2 tablespoons maple syrup or a low-carb sweetener (like stevia or monk fruit) to taste
- 1 teaspoon cinnamon
- 1/4 teaspoon nutmeg (optional)
- 1 tablespoon coconut oil or unsalted butter, melted
- *Optional*
  Greek yogurt or dairy-free yogurt for serving

DIRECTIONS

1. **Preheat Oven:** Preheat your oven to 350°F (175°C).
2. **Prepare Apples:** Core the apples, making sure to leave the bottom intact to hold the filling. You can use an apple corer or a knife to carefully remove the core.
3. **Make Filling:** In a mixing bowl, combine the chopped walnuts, raisins (if using), maple syrup (or sweetener), cinnamon, nutmeg (if using), and melted coconut oil (or butter). Mix until well combined.
4. **Stuff Apples:** Place the cored apples in a baking dish and fill each apple with the walnut mixture, packing it down gently.
5. **Bake:** Add a small amount of water (about 1/4 cup) to the bottom of the baking dish to help steam the apples. Cover the dish with foil and bake in the preheated oven for about 25-30 minutes, or until the apples are tender.
6. **Serve:** Remove from the oven and let cool slightly. Serve warm, optionally topped with a dollop of Greek yogurt or dairy-free yogurt.

Nutrition Information (Per Serving)

Calories	200
Protein	4g
Carbohydrates	30g
Dietary Fiber	5g
Sugars	15g
Fat	9g
Saturated Fat	2g

"Believe in your magic."

QUICK NOTES

TIPS FOR CUSTOMIZATION

- **Add Flavor:** Mix in a pinch of vanilla extract or almond extract for extra flavor.
- **Fruit Variations:** Substitute walnuts with pecans or almonds for different textures.
- **Sweetness Adjustments:** Adjust the sweetness based on the tartness of the apples and your personal preference.

Why is this recipe good for PCOS?

Baked apples are a great source of fiber and antioxidants, which help regulate blood sugar levels and promote satiety. The healthy fats from walnuts provide additional nutrients and support hormone balance. This warm and comforting dessert is nutritious, satisfying, and perfect for a healthy treat while managing PCOS.

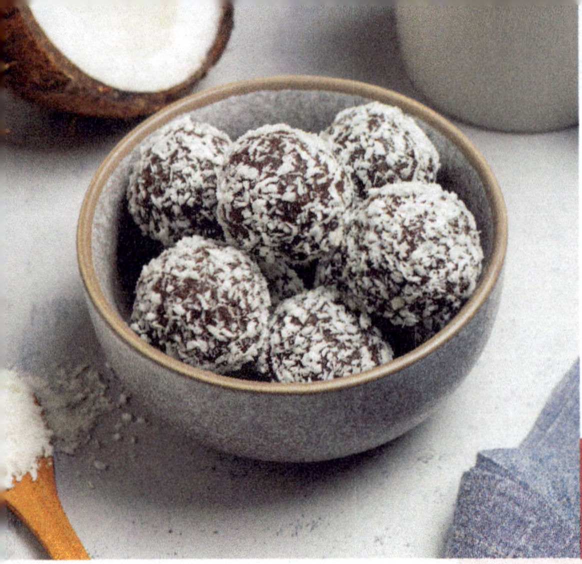

Lemon Coconut Energy Bites

SERVING SIZE
Serves 8 (2 bites per serving)

INGREDIENTS

- 1 cup rolled oats (gluten-free if needed)
- 1/2 cup unsweetened shredded coconut
- 1/2 cup almond butter (or any nut butter of your choice)
- 1/4 cup maple syrup or a low-carb sweetener (like stevia or monk fruit)
- Zest of 1 lemon
- Juice of 1 lemon
- 1/2 teaspoon vanilla extract
- Pinch of salt

DIRECTIONS

1. **Mix Ingredients:** In a large mixing bowl, combine the rolled oats, shredded coconut, almond butter, maple syrup (or sweetener), lemon zest, lemon juice, vanilla extract, and a pinch of salt. Mix until well combined and a sticky dough forms.
2. **Chill the Mixture:** Refrigerate the mixture for about 30 minutes to make it easier to handle.
3. **Form Bites:** Once chilled, use your hands to scoop out small portions of the mixture and roll them into bite-sized balls (about 1 inch in diameter).
4. **Coat (Optional):** If desired, roll the energy bites in additional shredded coconut for a decorative touch.
5. **Store:** Place the energy bites in an airtight container and store in the refrigerator for up to a week or in the freezer for longer storage.

Nutrition Information (Per Serving)

Calories	200
Protein	6g
Carbohydrates	24g
Dietary Fiber	4g
Sugars	5g
Fat	10g
Saturated Fat	2g

"You are the change-maker."

QUICK NOTES

TIPS FOR CUSTOMIZATION

- **Add Flavor:** Mix in a tablespoon of chia seeds or flaxseeds for added nutrition.
- **Nut Variations:** Substitute almond butter with peanut butter, cashew butter, or sunflower seed butter for variety.
- **Sweetness Adjustments:** Adjust the sweetness based on your preference and the tartness of the lemon.

Why is this recipe good for PCOS?

These lemon coconut energy bites are rich in healthy fats and fiber, which help regulate blood sugar levels and promote satiety. The combination of oats and nut butter provides sustained energy, making them a great snack option for women managing PCOS. This recipe is easy to prepare, nutritious, and perfect for a quick energy boost throughout the day.

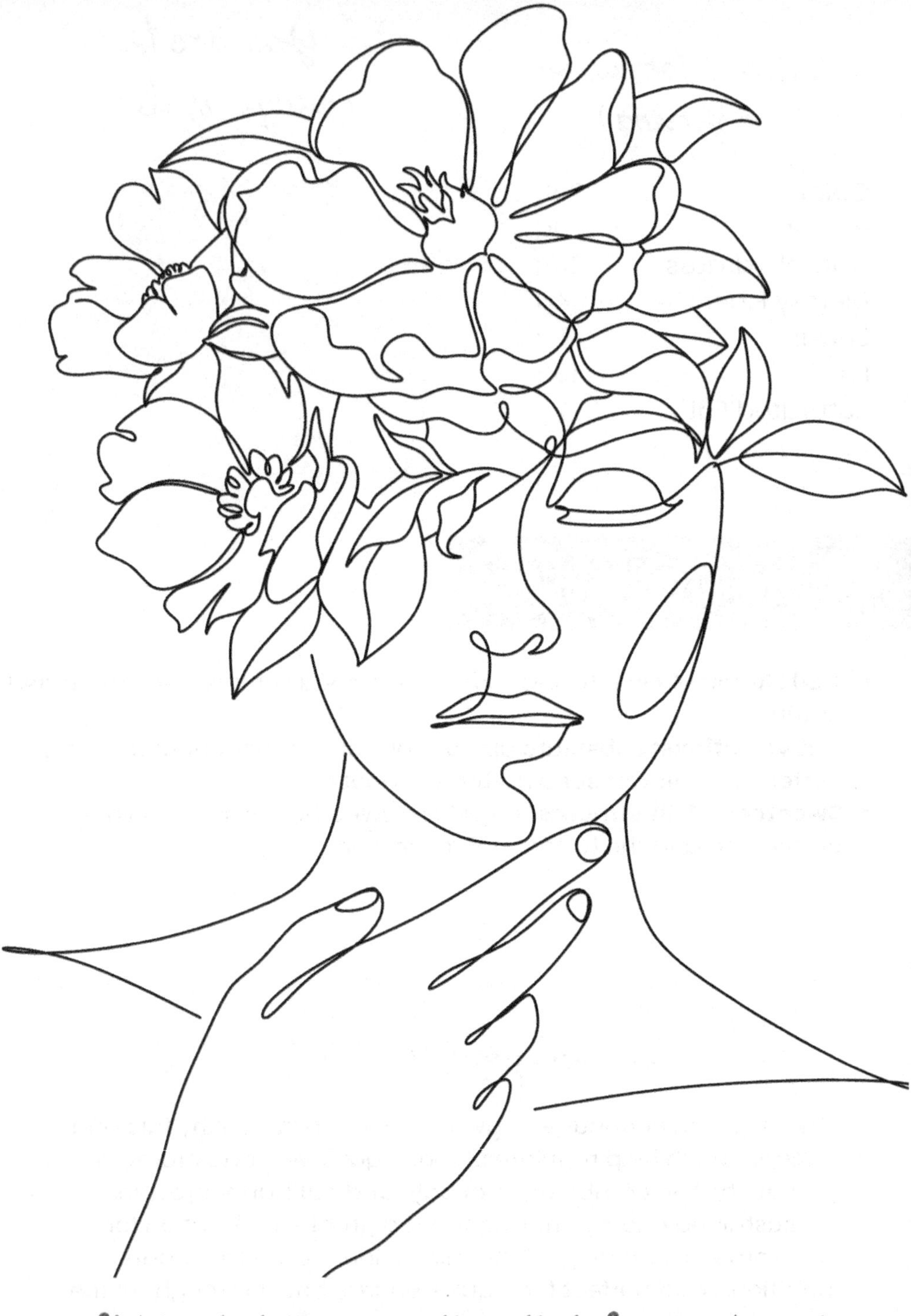

... I'd like to tell you something that I remind myself everyday -- You truly are strong and beautiful!

Chapter 11

Portion Control and Blood Sugar Hacks

Understanding Portion Control

Portion control is a crucial aspect of managing PCOS and maintaining a healthy weight. It involves being mindful of the amount of food you consume, which can help regulate blood sugar levels and prevent overeating. By understanding appropriate portion sizes, you can enjoy your favorite foods while still making choices that support your health.

Strategies for Managing Portion Sizes

- ***Use Smaller Plates and Bowls:***
  - Research shows that using smaller dishes can help you feel satisfied with smaller portions. This simple trick can reduce the likelihood of overeating.
- ***Measure Your Food:***
  - Initially, measuring your food can help you understand what a proper portion looks like. Use measuring cups or a food scale to get a sense of serving sizes for different foods.
- ***Practice Mindful Eating:***
  - Slow down and savor each bite. Pay attention to your hunger cues and stop eating when you feel satisfied, not stuffed. This practice can help you enjoy your food more and prevent overeating.
- ***Fill Half Your Plate with Vegetables:***
  - When preparing meals, aim to fill half your plate with non-starchy vegetables. This not only increases fiber intake but also helps control portion sizes for higher-calorie foods.
- ***Pre-Portion Snacks:***
  - Instead of eating directly from the package, portion out snacks into small containers or bags. This can help you avoid mindless snacking and keep your portions in check.
- ***Listen to Your Body:***
  - Tune in to your body's hunger and fullness signals. Eating when you're hungry and stopping when you're satisfied can help you maintain a healthy relationship with food.

Managing blood sugar levels is essential for women with PCOS, as insulin resistance can exacerbate symptoms. Here are some effective strategies to help balance your blood sugar while still enjoying treats:

Pair Carbohydrates with Protein and Healthy Fats:

- When consuming carbohydrates, pair them with protein and healthy fats to slow down digestion and prevent blood sugar spikes. For example, enjoy apple slices with almond butter or whole grain toast with avocado.

Choose High-Fiber Foods:

- Foods high in fiber, such as vegetables, whole grains, and legumes, can help stabilize blood sugar levels. Incorporate these foods into your meals and snacks for better blood sugar control.

Limit Refined Sugars and Processed Foods:

- Minimize your intake of refined sugars and highly processed foods, as they can lead to rapid spikes in blood sugar. Opt for whole, nutrient-dense foods instead.

Stay Hydrated:

- Drinking plenty of water throughout the day can help regulate blood sugar levels. Sometimes, thirst can be mistaken for hunger, leading to unnecessary snacking.

Incorporate Regular Physical Activity:

- Exercise can improve insulin sensitivity and help regulate blood sugar levels. Aim for at least 150 minutes of moderate-intensity exercise each week, incorporating both aerobic and strength-training activities.

Enjoy Treats Mindfully:

- When indulging in treats, practice moderation. Allow yourself to enjoy your favorite desserts or snacks, but be mindful of portion sizes. Savor each bite and enjoy the experience without guilt.

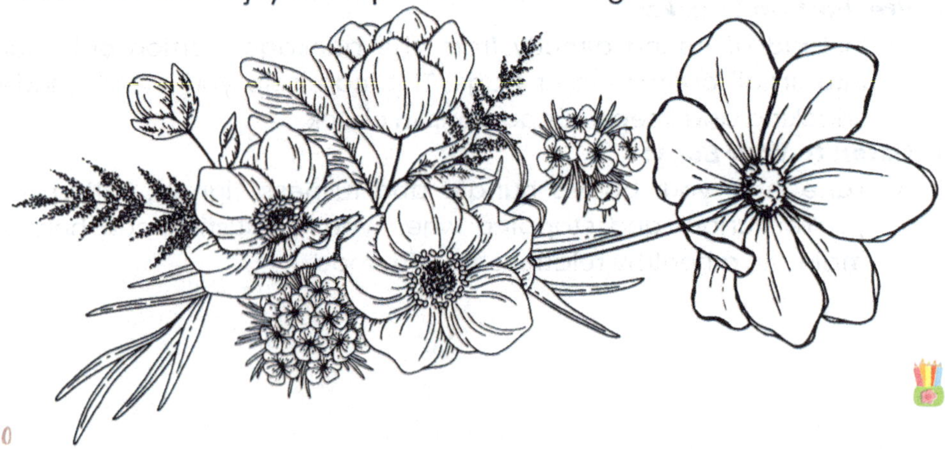

Chapter 12

Measurement

Measurement in Cooking

Accurate measurements are essential in cooking and baking, especially when it comes to creating healthy recipes that support your journey with PCOS. Understanding how to convert measurements can help you adapt recipes to fit your needs, ensuring that you maintain the right balance of ingredients for optimal nutrition. This chapter provides a handy guide for converting measurements commonly used in recipes, making it easier for you to prepare delicious meals.

Common Measurement Conversion

Volume Conversions

- 1 tablespoon (tbsp) = 3 teaspoons (tsp)
- 1/4 cup = 4 tablespoons
- 1/3 cup = 5 tablespoons + 1 teaspoon
- 1/2 cup = 8 tablespoons
- 1 cup = 16 tablespoons
- 1 pint = 2 cups
- 1 quart = 4 cups
- 1 gallon = 16 cups

Weight Conversions

- 1 ounce (oz) = 28 grams (g)
- 1 pound (lb) = 16 ounces = 454 grams
- 1 kilogram (kg) = 2.2 pounds.

Common Ingredient Conversions

- 1 cup of all-purpose flour = approximately 120 grams
- 1 cup of granulated sugar = approximately 200 grams
- 1 cup of brown sugar (packed) = approximately 220 grams
- 1 cup of rolled oats = approximately 90 grams
- 1 cup of cooked quinoa = approximately 185 grams
- 1 medium avocado = approximately 150 grams

- *Use the Right Tools*: Invest in a set of measuring cups and spoons for volume measurements, and a kitchen scale for weight measurements. This will help ensure accuracy in your cooking.

- *Level Off Dry Ingredients*: When measuring dry ingredients like flour or sugar, use a straight edge (like a knife) to level off the top of the measuring cup for an accurate measurement.

- *Pack Brown Sugar*: When measuring brown sugar, pack it firmly into the measuring cup to ensure you have the correct amount.

- *Liquid Measurements*: For liquid ingredients, use a clear measuring cup with measurement markings. Check the measurement at eye level to ensure accuracy.

- *Convert as Needed*: If a recipe calls for a different measurement than you have, use the conversion guide above to adjust accordingly. This will help you maintain the integrity of the recipe while accommodating your needs.

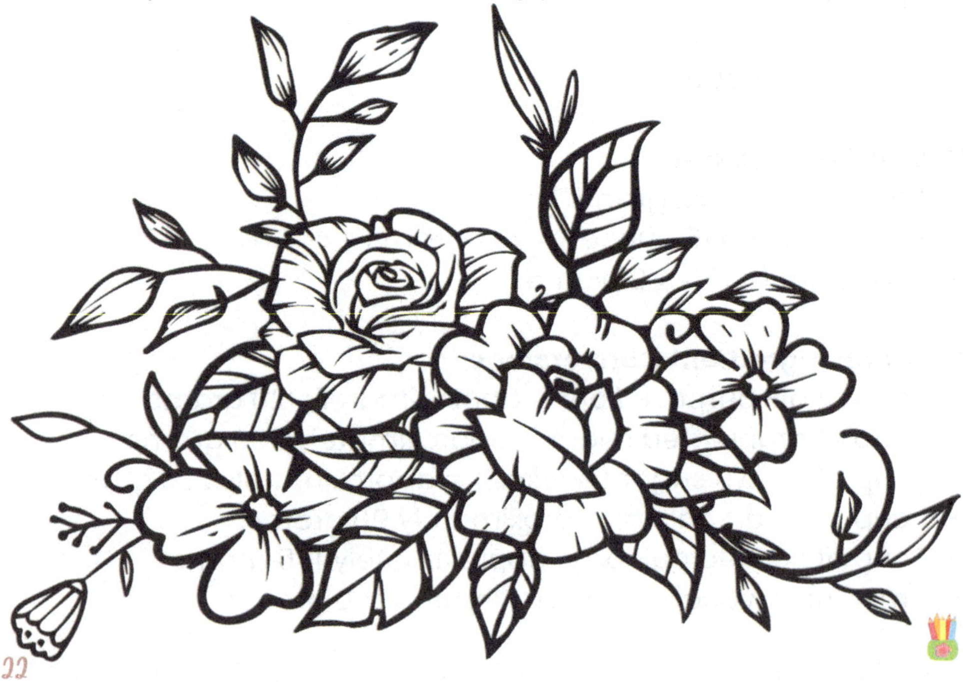

Chapter 13

Conclusion: Healing Together

Embracing the Journey

As we reach the end of this book, it's important to reflect on the journey we've taken together. Managing Polycystic Ovarian Syndrome (PCOS) can be challenging, but it is also an opportunity for growth, self-discovery, and empowerment. Through the recipes, tips, and insights shared in this book, I hope you feel equipped to take charge of your health and embrace a lifestyle that supports your well-being.

The Power of Nutrition

Nutrition is a powerful tool in managing PCOS. By focusing on whole, nutrient-dense foods and adopting a balanced approach to eating, you can positively impact your symptoms, regulate your cycle, and enhance your fertility. Remember, it's not about strict diets or deprivation; it's about making informed choices that nourish your body and soul.

Community and Support

You are not alone on this journey. Many women are navigating similar challenges, and together, we can create a supportive community. Share your experiences, celebrate your victories, and lean on each other for encouragement. Whether it's through online forums, local support groups, or friends and family, connecting with others can provide invaluable emotional support and motivation.

Mindset Matters

As you continue on your path, remember the importance of a positive mindset. Be kind to yourself and recognize that progress takes time. Celebrate small victories, and don't be discouraged by setbacks. Each step you take toward better health is a step in the right direction. Journaling your thoughts and feelings can be a powerful way to process your journey and maintain a positive outlook.

Moving Forward

As you move forward, keep the principles outlined in this book in mind. Embrace the 80/20 rule, make smart swaps, and practice portion control. Use the recipes as a guide to create meals that not only satisfy your cravings but also support your health. Remember that every meal is an opportunity to nourish your body and honor your journey.

Final Thoughts

In closing, I want to remind you that healing is a journey, not a destination. It's about finding balance, embracing your unique path, and making choices that align with your goals and values. You have the power to create a life filled with health, happiness, and fulfillment.

Thank you for allowing me to be a part of your journey. Together, we can heal, thrive, and support one another in managing PCOS through nutrition and self-care. Here's to your health and happiness!

Thank you very much!

Dear Cysters,

Thank you for being a part of this journey toward better health and wellness! Your support means the world to me, and I hope that the recipes and insights in "Nurse's Guide to PCOS Diet Without Deprivation" have empowered you on your path.

If you enjoyed the cookbook, I would be incredibly grateful if you could take a moment to leave a review on Amazon. Your feedback not only helps me improve but also supports other women looking for guidance in managing PCOS.
You can leave your review by following the link or by scanning the QR code below:

go.binnovatedigital.com/pcosrecipes1

Thank you for your support, and remember, we are all in this together!

With love and gratitude,

Giselle ♡

Made in the USA
Monee, IL
03 November 2026

67387160R00075